Let My People Breathe!

Unmasking the Mask Controversy

With Science and Scripture

Surgical and Cloth Masks Don't Work to "Reduce the Spread" – a review of the science and a return to FREEDOM!

Dr. Jerry Scheidbach (Doctor of Theological Studies-DTS)

Sarah Green (Certified Physician Assistant-PA-C)

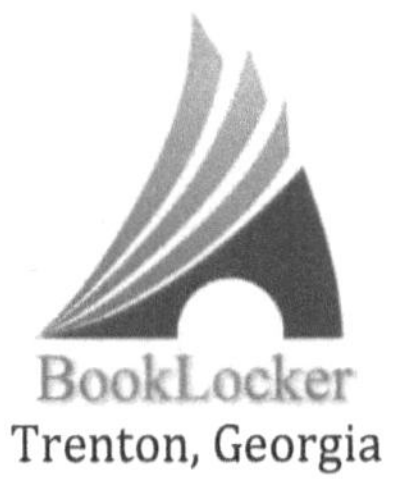

BookLocker

Trenton, Georgia

About the Authors

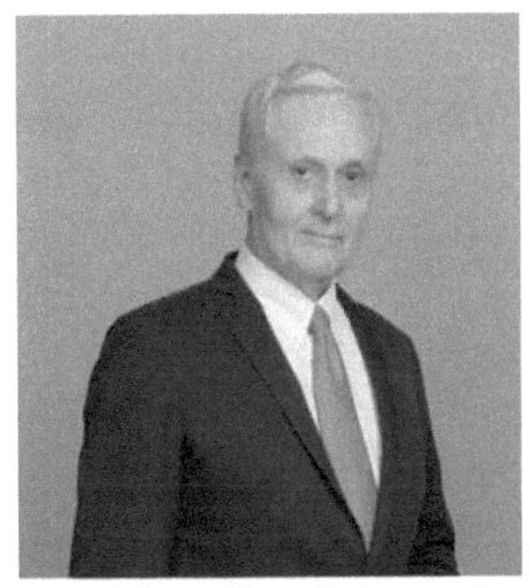

The author, Dr. Jerry Scheidbach (DTS), pastors Lighthouse Baptist Church in Santa Maria, CA, hosts the *Brain Massage®* radio/podcast, and livestreams *Comfort & Counsel For the Present Distress.* He serves as Evangelist Dr. Benny Beckum's executive editor for *The Intercessor* magazine, and is honored to preach Prayer Conferences with him. Dr. Scheidbach is an invited guest to many pulpits in the US, and is often asked to conduct prophecy conferences (US, RU, FJ, MX, CA). He has authored several books: *God's War, The New Cart Church, Kingdom Power by Prayer and Fasting, My Notes On the Visions of Daniel,* among others. He served as president of Eurasia Baptist Bible College, headquartered in Moscow, RU, and as professor of theology for Pacific Coast Baptist Bible College (now Heartland Baptist College, OK), and as guest lecturer at Lancaster Baptist College and Pacific Baptist College, both in CA.

Dr. Scheidbach received his Thg (equivalent to an AA) and BA from Pacific Coast Baptist Bible College, CA, his MA from Liberty University, VA (magna cum laude), and his Doctor of Theological Studies (DTS) from Bethany Seminary, AL (summa cum laude). He was introduced to biblical Hebrew at Temple Beth Torah, Ventura, CA, and studied conversational Hebrew using the Pimsleur Language Course. He has served in full time Christian ministry for over 50 years (started pastoring at 20 yrs old), including six years as principal of Baptist Christian Schools, Norwalk, CA. He has served his current pastorate for twenty-seven years.

You can reach Dr. Scheidbach through his website: godswar2020.com, by email at pastor@baptistlighthouse.org, or by text or phone at 805.714.0786.

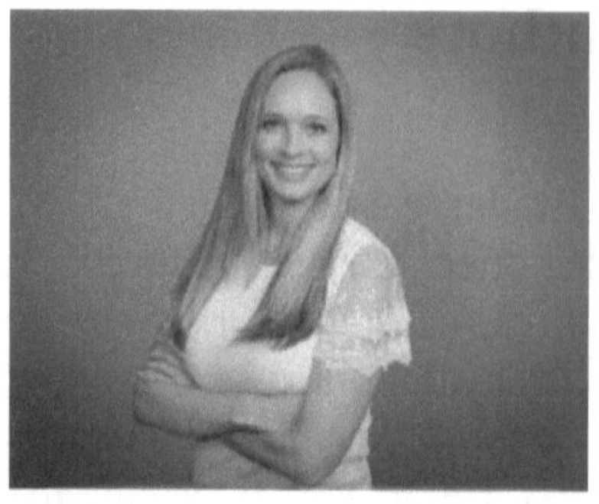

Contributing author Sarah Green is a certified Physician Assistant (PA-C). Born and reared in Santa Barbara, CA., she remembers wanting to work in the medical field from childhood. Sarah completed her undergraduate work at Cal State Channel Islands in Camarillo, CA. In her anatomy class, she met a fellow student studying to be a Physician Assistant. She made further inquiries and felt strongly that Physician Assistant was the field of medicine that fit her goals.

After graduating from the Western University of Health Sciences in Pomona, CA, Sarah joined the staff of Santa Barbara Cottage Hospital, serving in their trauma/surgery department. While employed there, Sarah explored gynecology (GYN), weight control, and esthetics. After nine years at Cottage Hospital, Sarah moved to Nipomo and accepted a position at Dignity Health, working in their Urgent Care center in Orcutt, CA. She was employed with Dignity Health for two years.

During her time at Dignity Health, Orcutt Urgent Care, COVID broke out. Sarah noticed that although she was hearing and reading about how destructive it was and that hospitals were overrun, her urgent care center was like a ghost town. Whereas before COVID, Orcutt Urgent Care attended to over 100 patients a day, after COVID, it dropped to about 10 per day. Furthermore, she noticed the hospitals were empty, although news outlets kept reporting they were overflowing. Things didn't add up. And it didn't take long before Sarah realized the media was pushing a false narrative about this pandemic, and she was not buying it. After intensive deep-dive research, she confirmed that the narrative pushed by the media and the medical establishment was not true. Sarah knew something was very wrong!

Then came the vaccines! Sarah's medical training told her a vaccine usually requires five years of trials. Having a vaccine-injured son heightened her concerns about rushing a vaccine into public use. Additionally, she was concerned because the technology used for this vaccine was something new and unproven. Sarah refused to take "the jab."

After the vaccine rollout, Sarah started seeing a spike in COVID cases and patients experiencing vaccine injury symptoms. She treated her patients with medications she used when she got COVID that helped her recover quickly. Patients thanked her, saying how much better they felt after their treatment. Dignity Health objected that Sarah was not following "protocol." She was scolded! Convinced the COVID treatment protocol insisted upon by her employer was wrong for her patients and determined to provide them the best and most effective care she could, Sarah left Dignity Health and never returned. She was relieved, supposing she would be free from seeing COVID patients.

But GOD had another plan for Sarah. A flood of opportunities came her way to help those suffering from COVID and vaccine-related injuries. The treatments she prescribed were helping her patients, but soon she began to notice the medication best suited to their needs was becoming increasingly difficult to come by. Sarah discovered that even the pharmacies had been politicized. For the first time in her career, pharmacies refused to fill her prescriptions. It took some research and several hours of phone calls, but Sarah found a way to help her patients.

Over the past year and a half, Sarah has treated over 2,000 COVID patients. She considers it to have been the biggest blessing in her life. Because of her faithfulness to her oath as a medical professional and commitment to her patients, GOD used her knowledge to help so many who were desperate and in need of care. Today, Sarah enjoys professional and personal satisfaction in her work and deep gratitude to her Lord Jesus for His continued guidance in her medical practice.

©Sarah Green

Contact Sarah Green through her website: (Central Coast Alternative Therapeutics & Rejuvenation) ccatr.us (under construction as of 3/16/23, launch date 2023), or call her office at 805.619.7515.

Special Acknowledgement

Christine (Chris) Pace began her career as a CNA, went to nursing school, and became an LVN. She continued her studies to obtain her RN license and served 35 years as a medical professional. She gives God praise for honoring her with the privilege to serve her Lord by loving and ministering to His people in physical and emotional need. Her areas of service included Obstetrics, New Born Nursery, Pediatrics, Home Health, wound care specialist, Intensive Care Unit, Emergency Room, medical-surgical nursing, outpatient surgery/recovery, and geriatric liaison. Chris continues today to serve as a patient advocate for those God brings along her path and takes it as her greatest honor to serve under the "Great Physician" as His blessed assistant.

When Dr. Jerry Scheidbach asked Chris to review his manuscript she carefully examined his work and wrote the following: "Thank you for sending *Let my people Breathe*. It is very well done Jerry, full of true and insightful info! I found absolutely nothing to change or add to! You did very thorough research and your medical information was exact! ... The medical mask info you laid out is Medical Science 101! After serving in that field over 30 years, I have struggled greatly with the info provided/mandated by our government and even more with the compliance! People are fearful of losing their jobs, their income potential, their reputations, their health—their material "things"! So many have been duped! Thank you, Jerry, for speaking the truth! May God richly bless you as you provide His truth to His people Brother!"

Table of Contents

Preface/Foreword

Normally, a preface would provide background believed helpful to give context for the content that follows. All that is needed in that way is incorporated into the text of this book. I will use this space to discuss the extent and method of my research.

Virtually every scientific research paper provides a statement regarding the type of research being done and the method used by the authors. What follows approximates a disclosure of my research extent and methods. For a full explanation, see SUPPLEMENTAL material and read the introduction to *Let My People Breathe (RESEARCH NOTES)*. In summary, my research type fits the category of a *review of the literature* on the subject of mask efficacy. As for methods, I zeroed in on the 49 scientific articles presented by investigative reporter, Russell Falcon, purporting to prove masks are efficacious to "stop the spread" of a virus, and in the work of vetting these articles, I expanded my research into supporting data and technical articles. The methods employed are detailed in the introduction of *Let My People Breathe (RESEARCH NOTES)*. (Of particular interest will be my notes on the issue of bias.)

There are four supplementary research folders available online to all who purchase this book. The four folders are titled as follows: OR—Opposition Research - Research Opposing My Thesis (597 research articles); OAI—Other Articles of Interest (135 research articles); SE—Supporting Evidence - Research Supporting My Thesis (135 research articles); and TECH—Technical Articles Related To Mask Use (97 research articles), for a total of 964 research articles examined for this book.

My focus was on scientific research that proved masks were effective to "stop the spread." For that reason, I concentrated on evidence that opposed my thesis. So the largest folder is named *OR—Opposition Research - Research Opposing My Thesis* and contains well over half of the total number of articles I vetted for this book. The OR folder contains a PDF copy of every research article I vetted while researching the claims made in the 49 studies presented by investigative journalist Russell Falcon in his article titled *Do face masks work? Here are 49 scientific studies that explain why they do,* August 7, 2021, updated September 17, 2021. I refer to these collectively as the *Falcon 49.* In this folder, you will find a PDF copy of each article examined. The folder is so large it had to be broken into seven zip files: OR.1, OR.2, etc., through OR.7. Accompanying these folders, the reader will find an introduction to my research methods, a table of codes and abbreviations, and over 2000 pages of research notes, titled *Let My People Breathe (RESEARCH NOTES)* — the font size is set at 20 pts for ease of use; at a standard 12 pt. font, the page count is 884 pages. Also included in this folder is a chronological table of the articles vetted.

The next folder is titled *SE—Supporting Evidence - Research Supporting My Thesis.* It contains 135 articles that prove masks do not work to stop the spread of a virus. The fact that the opposing research includes 597 articles and supporting research includes only 135 does not mean there are fewer studies supporting than opposing the use of masks. The larger number of articles opposing my thesis is owing to the fact that I went out of my way to carefully examine the opposition to my thesis. It is also somewhat reflective of the fact that studies favoring masks have multiplied, and studies exposing masks as ineffective have greatly declined in the politicized environment surrounding COVID-19.

OAI—Other Articles of Interest comes next, including another 135 articles that for the most part offer information related to the topic of this book, mask efficacy, but were not directly or indirectly referenced in my vetting of the *Falcon 49.*

Finally, the last folder is *TECH—Technical Articles Related to the Mask Issue,* where the reader will find another 97 articles addressing technical aspects of my research: what is focal length in photography, offering technical information regarding the use of photography to measure particles, and studies explaining the movement of particles, etc.; characterization of particle size, distribution of exhaled droplets, etc.; what is an RCT, what is an observational study, what is the scientific method, and so on.

Contact Dr. Scheidbach for the coupon code to download the SUPPLEMENTAL Material free with proof of purchase. Go to www.godswar2020.com and use the contact email form.

Dear Reader, do your own research and draw your own conclusions. The truth will speak for itself; an honest student will hear what truth says; and as Jesus promised, the truth shall make you FREE (John 8:32).

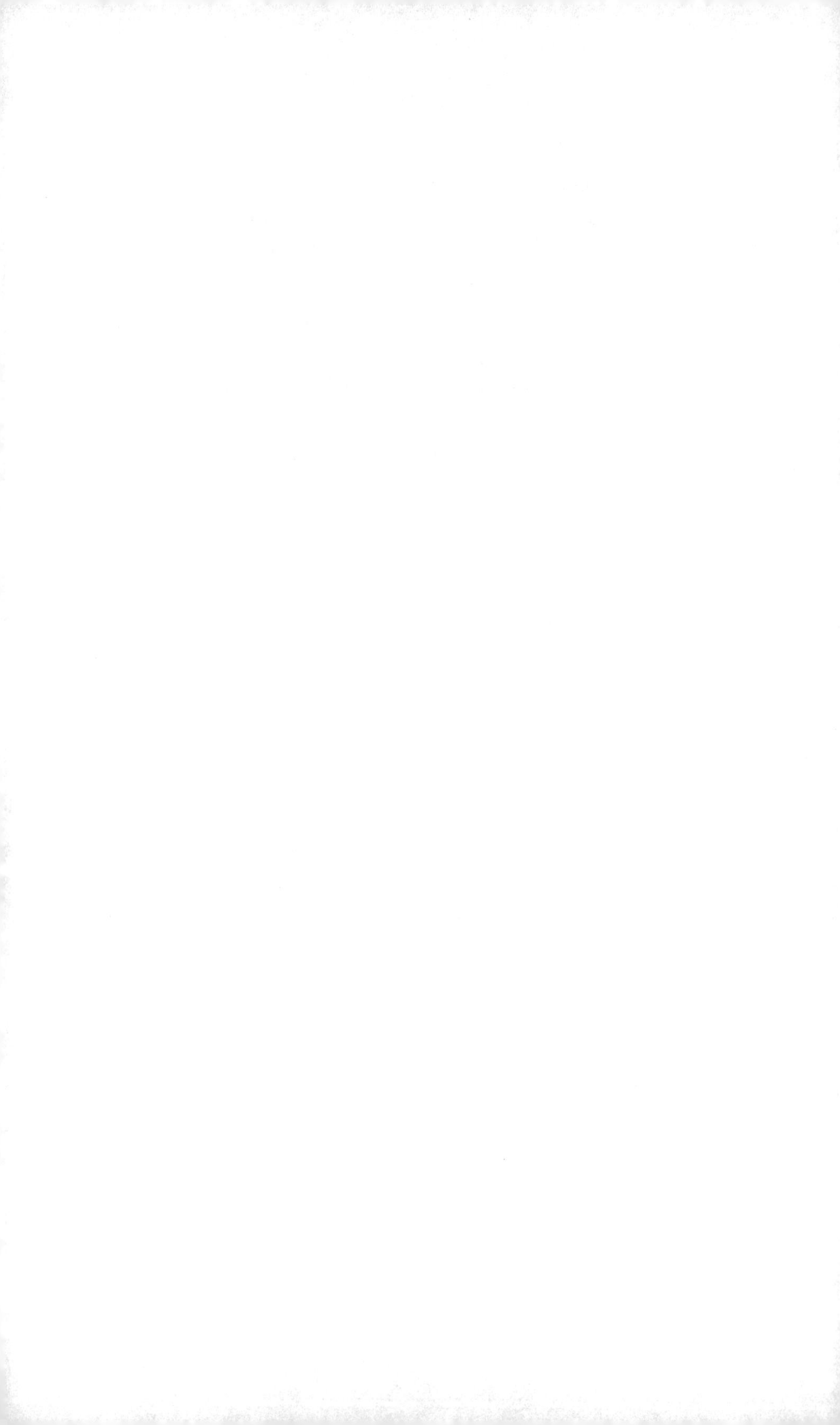

Part One:
Follow the Science

Chapter One:
What Science Are We Supposed to Follow?

We are told to follow the science. *Some* medical doctors say we must wear masks to stop the spread! Others disagree! Here is a link to one article that cites 49 studies supporting masks as a way to control the spread of any virus.[1]

(https://www.kxan.com/news/coronavirus/do-face-masks-work-here-are-49-scientific-studies-that-explain-why-they-do/)

But here is another link to research that cites fifty scientific studies showing proof masks "do nothing to prevent the spread of illness."[2]

(https://www.dailyveracity.com/2021/07/26/over-50-scientific-studies-conclude-masks-do-nothing-to-prevent-the-spread-of-illness-so-why-do-people-keep-claiming-they-work/)

How can we follow the science if scientists disagree about what the science says?

---

[1] Falcon, Russell, KXAN—Austin, TX, *Do face masks work? Here are 49 scientific studies that explain why they do,* August 7, 2021, updated September 17, 2021, published by KXAN, an NBC news affiliate. [ONLINE: https://www.kxan.com/news/coronavirus/do-face-masks-work-here-are-49-scientific-studies-that-explain-why-they-do/ — 11/17/22] For PDF, see Doc. Folder OR - FN01.00.00.00.00. I have carefully examined every one of these research papers and not one of them proves masks protect the wearer or the community from virions in the size range of SARS-CoV-2, which are 40-170 nanometers (nm) in diameter, or against droplets that are <300 nanometers. Nor do these research articles provide proof masks provide adequate protection against infection from droplets that are ≥300 nanometers to ≤5 μm (5000 nm).

[2] Daily Veracity, Staff, July 26, 2021, Over 50 Scientific Studies Conclude Masks Do Nothing to Prevent the Spread of Illness, So Why Do People Keep Claiming They Work? [ONLINE: https://www.dailyveracity.com/2021/07/26/over-50-scientific-studies-conclude-masks-do-nothing-to-prevent-the-spread-of-illness-so-why-do-people-keep-claiming-they-work/ — 9/22/22]. For PDF, see Doc. Folder OR - FN02. "The vast majority of gold-standard scientific research compiled over multiple decades, conclude masks are completely ineffective at preventing the spread of respiratory illness." See also Doc. Folder SE - SE035 for 150+ studies showing masks are ineffective to protect from a virus.

Why is there so much confusion about this?

For almost 100 years, western medical science has agreed that masks do not provide adequate protection against viral infection. Suddenly, all of that changed! But no one told us why!

As late as February 2020, Fauci sent an email to Obama-appointed Health and Human Services Secretary, Sylvia Burwell, responding to a question she asked about wearing masks for protection against viral infection. He recommended against it because, as he explained, "The typical mask you buy in the drug store is not really effective in keeping out virus, which is small enough to pass through the material."[3] But by June 2020, Fauci changed his mind and began recommending everyone wear the very kind of mask he told Burwell is "not really effective in keeping out virus." Indeed, Fauci became a mask zealot, insisting everyone must wear them.[4] What happened?

Dr. Fauci was asked why he did not recommend public use of masks at the beginning of the pandemic. He explained that he feared it would trigger panic buying creating a shortage that would make them unavailable to health care workers.[5] Whatever his motivations, Fauci admitted he lied. Even his lie was a lie! Concern about shortages was not on his mind when he told Sylvia Burwell to not bother wearing one because they do not provide protection against a virus. He explained why he lied to us when he said we

---

[3] Fauci, email to HHS Secretary Burwell, Feb. 2020 [ONLINE: https://nationalfile.com/fauci-told-former-obama-admin-official-in-a-private-email-dont-wear-a-mask/] For PDF, see Doc. Folder OAI93. Here is the full text of Dr. Fauci's email referenced in this article: "Sylvia: Masks are really for infected people to prevent them from spreading infection to people who are not infected rather than protecting uninfected people from acquiring infection. The typical mask you buy in the drug store is not really effective in keeping out virus, which is small enough to pass through the material. It might, however, provide some slight benefit in keep [sic] out gross droplets if someone coughs or sneezes on you. I do not recommend that you wear a mask, particularly since you are going to a very low risk location. Your instincts are correct, [sic—;] money is best spent on medical countermeasures such as diagnostics and vaccines. Safe travels."

[4] Kelley, Alexandra, *Fauci: why the public wasn't told to wear masks when the coronavirus pandemic began,* The Hill, Changing America, June 16, 2020 [ONLINE: https://thehill.com/changing-america/well-being/prevention-cures/502890-fauci-why-the-public-wasnt-told-to-wear-masks/ — 9/22/22]. For PDF, see Doc. Folder: OAI36. See also OAI35.

[5] IBID. Kelley, Alexandra.

should not bother wearing them, but why did he lie to Burwell when he told her they don't protect against a virus?

Did some new science emerge that overturned almost 100 years of science-based western medical consensus regarding masks? No! Fauci has never directed us to any study that proved western scientists had been wrong about masks for about 100 years, or that he was wrong when he advised Burwell not to wear one.

The rationale for the mysterious Fauci flip-flop on masks will be discussed later. For now, it's not at all hard to see why there is so much confusion about this, and about a great many other things that went on, and still go on with this pandemic.

"God is not the author of confusion." [6] James said out of confusion arises "every evil work."[7]

What science should we follow?

Mr. Anderson, writing for *City Journal*, examined the evidence on both sides and explained: "Medical studies on masking ... fall into one of two categories: observational studies or randomized controlled trials, dubbed RCTs."[8] Indeed, each of the more than 700 research studies and articles on masks that I examined may be characterized as either an RCT or some species of an observational study.

---

[6] 1Corinthians 14:33

[7] James 3:16

[8] Anderson, Jeffery H., *Do Masks Work? A review of the evidence*, City Journal, August 11, 2021. [Online: https://www.city-journal.org/do-masks-work-a-review-of-the-evidence#.YRSMsaJRXXk.twitter]. For PDF, see Doc. Folder SE037. Mr. Anderson opened his article by quoting a Tweet from then surgeon general Jerome Adams on February 29, 2020: "Seriously people—STOP BUYING MASKS! They are NOT effective in preventing general public from catching #Coronavirus." This is an excellent article, thoroughly documented, and well written. He observed what I did in my own research: "It is striking how much the CDC, in marshalling [sic] evidence to justify its revised mask guidance, studiously avoids mentioning randomized controlled trials." For an update to this article, see *Masks Still Don't Work: More than two year on, the best scientific evidence says that masks don't stop Covid—and public health officials continue to ignore it,* August 8, 2022 [ONLINE: https://www.city-journal.org/masks-still-dont-work] For PDF, see Doc. Folder OAl37.

Dr. Fauci testified before the House about use of hydroxychloroquine (HCQ) as early treatment for COVID-19. He explained that randomized controlled trials (RCTs) are the gold standard of medical research,[9] and that there were no randomized placebo-controlled trials supporting the use of HCQ for COVID-19. Yet there are many qualified RCTs that show masks are not effective to protect against a virus.[10] In the case of masks, Fauci ignores the science. We might ask Dr. Fauci for clarity on when, exactly, we should follow the science?

The highest paid bureaucrat in the U.S. (more than $400k per year), and reputed virology expert, Dr. Anthony Fauci, said,

---

[9] House Coronavirus Hearing, July 31, 2020, Transcript: [ONLINE: https://www.rev.com/blog/transcripts/dr-fauci-hydroxychloroquine-statement-transcript-house-coronavirus-hearing-july-31 — 9/22/22]. For PDF, see Doc. Folder OAI39. Fauci asserted no "randomized placebo-controlled trials, which is the gold standard of determining if something is effective," had shown any efficacy by hydroxychloroquine. Curious, this same thing may be said of mask efficacy against virus and yet Fauci ignores that fact in his recommendations regarding them. The reverse might be charged against me, that I support use of HCQ for COVID-19 treatment even though it had no support from RCTs for use against COVID-19, but reject masks on the basis there are no RCTs that support them. First, there were no RCTs testing the efficacy of HCQ as a treatment for COVID-19, but there were many other studies that showed its effectiveness in treating similar issues. Second, there are many RCTs that show positively that masks are not effective to protect against virus infection. There are no RCTs that show HCQ is ineffective for treatment against COVID-19. Finally, as early as October 5, 2020, a study published in pubmed.gov website by the National Center for Biotechnology Information (NCBI), National Library of Medicine (NLM), within the auspices of the National Institutes of Health (NIH), NIH being the organization within which Fauci's NIAID operates, says "HCQ was found to be consistently effective against COVID-19 when provided early in the outpatient setting. It was also found to be overall effective in inpatient studies." The article is titled: *Hydroxychloroquine is effective, and consistently so when provided early, for COVID-19: a systematic review,* by authors C. Prodromos (Illinois Sports Medicine and Orthopedic Center, Glenview, IL, USA, and T. Rumschlag, Foundation for Orthopaedics and Regenerative Medicine, Glenview, IL, USA. There are no declared conflicts of interest, and no disclaimers. As for Ivermectin, the same pubmed.gov published a study that found Ivermectin effective in the treatment of COVID-19 patients: [ONLINE: https://www.ncbi.nlm.nih.gov/pmc/articles/PMC7709596/ — 11/17/22]. For PDF, see Doc. Folder OAI94.

[10] IBID. *Daily Veracity …* [ONLINE: https://www.dailyveracity.com/2021/07/26/over-50-scientific-studies-conclude-masks-do-nothing-to-prevent-the-spread-of-illness-so-why-do-people-keep-claiming-they-work/ — 9/22/22]. See the statement regarding RCTs, and Bin-Reza et al. (2012) in which 17 RCTs were examined and none supported masks as efficacious to protect against a virus. My own research involves examination of highly technical data derived from bona-fide scientific experiments that prove conclusively that masks do not provide adequate protection from virus transmission or contagion. See *Let My People Breathe: Research Notes* available as a free download at https://www.brainmassage.net —> Resources —> Let My People Breathe.

"Attacks on me, quite frankly, are attacks on science."[11] Maybe, in his mind, since he *is* science, following him is following science?

Another thing you must keep in mind when researching the science on masks is this — the statements of scientists are not science. Science is the hard work of research and experimentation that support scientists' statements.

At the outset of our examination of the question *which science should we follow,* I think we can begin by saying—*not Fauci.*

There is a rule found in the Bible that we are to "try the spirits" because there are many liars in the world.[12] When someone intentionally lies we know what spirit they are of: "Ye are of your father the devil ... When he speaketh a lie, he speaketh of his own: for he is a liar, and the father of it."[13]

What are Observational Studies and RCTs?

<u>Observational Studies</u> include anecdotal evidence—stories about someone's personal experience—or observations based on more or less loosely conducted experiments. They can be useful to consider whether a claim warrants closer examination, but these studies have not been well respected among serious scientists when used to make claims asserted to be supported by *science.* Among the reasons such studies are not respected as providing scientific proof is how easy it is to massage the results into conformity with prevailing bias. Also they are susceptible to what are called *confounders,* which are alternate explanations for the results obtained. Finally, it's practically impossible to replicate

---

[11]Porterfield, Carlie, Forbes Staff, Forbes, *Dr. Fauci On GOP Criticism: 'Attacks On Me, Quite Frankly, Are Attacks On Science"* see Crucial Quote [ONLINE: https://www.forbes.com/sites/carlieporterfield/2021/06/09/fauci-on-gop-criticism-attacks-on-me-quite-frankly-are-attacks-on-science/?sh=6cd3ca4b4542 — 9/22/22] For PDF see Doc. Folder: OAI.40

[12] 1John 4:1, "Beloved, believe not every spirit, but try the spirits whether they are of God: because many false prophets are gone out into the world." See also the warning of Paul in 1Timothy 4:1, "Now the Spirit speaketh expressly, that in the latter times some shall depart from the faith, giving heed to seducing spirits, and doctrines of devils."

[13] John 8:44

these studies and provide consistent outcomes. Observational studies depend too heavily upon correlation. Every trained scientist knows mere correlation does not prove causation. I'll illustrate!

The *Canadian Medical Association Journal* published an article purporting to present evidence that masks protect against the spread of COVID-19. [14] The conclusion was derived from the story of a COVID-19 positive airline passenger who wore a mask on a flight and none of the other 200+ passengers subsequently tested positive. However, the observed effect (*no other passenger tested positive for COVID*) was not necessarily caused by the correlated event (*one COVID positive passenger wore a mask on that flight*). Let me explain.

First, we don't know what would have happened if that passenger had not worn a mask. Second, this story might have as easily been offered to prove the efficacy of the filtration system of the airplane. Perhaps whatever virions (infectious virus particles) escaped the mask were captured by the plane's highly efficient filters. Third, this was not a scientific experiment, with controls in place to protect the study from such confounders, and it does not provide for replication in order to prove the validity of any conclusions derived from it. The above by no means exhausts all the reasons this story cannot be taken seriously as scientific proof regarding anything about masks, but I think what is presented here is sufficient to show why observational studies are not depended upon to establish scientific conclusions.

Nevertheless, the above story was offered as a serious medical study by a respected medical journal, and it has been repeatedly used to support recommendations for the use of masks to protect against viral spread. It's alarming that the prestigious *Canadian*

---

[14] Schwartz, K., et. al. *Lack of COVID-19 transmission on an international flight,* cmajGROUP (Canadian Medical Association Journal), April 14, 2020 [ONLINE: https://www.cmaj.ca/content/192/15/E410 — 9/21/22] For PDF, see Doc. Folder OR - FN01.05.00.00.00.

Medical Association Journal would publish such an account as if it was serious science. Later, I will show how western science has shifted from insistence upon empirical observations based on experiments designed specifically to eliminate confounders to what amounts to the stuff silly superstitions are made of.

<u>Let's talk about the RCT</u>. The gold standard for scientific medical research is the Randomized Controlled Trial (RCT). A proper RCT is carefully constructed and conducted with a high degree of professional integrity. A good RCT scrupulously follows the *scientific method*.[15] The RCT is respected because properly conducted research of this kind will minimize confounders, and produce results that can be replicated by anyone else following the methods used. Western medical science has insisted on RCTs as the basis for supporting science based medical claims regarding causation since Austin Bradford Hill (1897-1991) conceived it in 1948.[16] Only recently have western scientists begun to pull away from Bradford's model and his insistence upon rigorous experimentation as they move toward the more loosely constructed observational science models favored by eastern medical traditions.

Follow True Science!

Here is the first thing you need to know when following the science. Fact: no properly constructed and conducted RCTs

---

[15] Wright, Gavin, author, Lavery, Tresa, edt. assistant, DEFINITION *scientific method*. WhatIs.com, [ONLINE https://www.techtarget.com/whatis/ definition/scientific-method — 9/21/22] For PDF, see Doc. Folder TECH93. Curiously, the authors include Darwin as a contributor to the scientific method as one who was "known for using multiple communication channels to share his conclusions"? What has that to do with the *scientific method* for ascertaining proof for a hypothesis? Almost no recent publication can be trusted to not in one way or another promote the establishment narrative. Hundreds of reputable scientists have walked away from Darwin ([ONLINE: https://newspunch.com/hundreds-scientists-question-darwins-theory-evolution/ — 9/21/22] For PDF, see Doc. Folder OAI95.

[16] British Medical Journal, London, *Streptomycin Treatment of Pulmonary Tuberculosis: A Medical Research Council Investigation,* The James Lind Library, October 30, 1948 [ONLINE: https://www.jameslindlibrary.org/medical-research-council-1948b/ — 9/20/22]. For PDF see Documentation Supplement: Doc. Folder OAI32.

support the masks Fauci and friends recommend to protect anyone from transmitting or contracting a viral infection.[17]

A quick look at the Cochrane controversy:

Cochrane is a trusted source for medical professionals providing analysis and summaries of the best evidence from biomedical research, "without interference from commercial and financial interests, and is the leading global advocate for evidence-based health care."[18] This reputable and highly respected source for clinical and biomedical guidance recently published the results of their own review of the science on the question of mask efficacy against COVID-19. Under *Key messages:* the Cochrane review stated: "We are uncertain whether wearing masks or N95/P2 respirators helps to slow the spread of respiratory viruses based on the studies we assessed."[19] In other words, Cochrane could not

---

[17] Rancourt, Denis, PhD., *Masks don't work — a review of the science relevant to Covid-19 social policy,* The Wall Will Fall, June 23, 2020 [ONLINE: https://thewallwillfall.org/2020/06/23/masks-dont-work-a-review-of-science-relevant-to-covid-19-social-policy/] For PDF, see Doc. Folder SE012.00.00.00. "No RCT study with verified outcome shows a benefit for HCW [Health Care Workers] or community members in households to wearing a mask or respirator. There is no such study. There are no exceptions." Even those in favour of masks know there are no RCTs that support them. In *Let My People Breathe (Research Notes)* I repeatedly documented corroborating statements in articles/studies that supported mask use. Here are only three of many examples that could be cited: 1. Leung, et. al. in an article titled *Mask wearing to complement social distancing and save lives during COVID-19,* said "there have not been randomised controlled trials to show the efficacy of mask wearing" [ONLINE: https://theunion.org/sites/default/files/2020-09/IJTLD%20June%200244%20Leung%20FINAL.pdf]. For PDF, see Doc. Folder OR - FN01.22.00.00.00. 2. Trish Greenhalgh, et. al. in *Masks for all: The science says yes,* after telling us no RCTs have been conducted to test efficacy against SARS-CoV-2 virus, writes: "RCTs of mask-wearing to prevent other diseases (such as influenza or tuberculosis) have tended to show a small effect which in many studies was not statistically significant." [ONLINE: https://www.fast.ai/2020/04/13/masks-summary/]. For PDF, see Doc. Folder OR - FN01.38.00.03.25L. 3. Huang, et. al., in *An evidence review of face masks against COVID-19* said, "WE SHOULD NOT BE SURPRISED TO FIND THAT THERE IS NO RCT FOR THE IMPACT OF MASKS ON COMMUNITY TRANSMISSION OF ANY RESPIRATORY INFECTION IN A PANDEMIC." [ONLINE: https://www.pnas.org/doi/10.1073/ pnas.2014564118]. For PDF, see Doc. Folder OR - FN01.38.00.03.00.

[18] Spira, Beny, *Cochrane Ends the Masking Rage,* Brownstone, Brownstone Institute Articles, March 9, 2023 [ONLINE: https://brownstone.org/articles/cochrane-ends-the-masking-rage/ — 3/14/23] For PDF, see Doc Folder SE038.

[19] Jefferson T, Dooley L, et al., *Do physical measures such as hand-washing or wearing masks stop or slow down the spread of respiratory viruses?* Cochrane, January 30, 2023 [ONLINE: https-

find support for the assertion that masks provide protection to the public from the spread of COVID-19 although they evaluated all the literature up through 2022.

What Cochrane found in this latest review (see above) reconfirmed an earlier December 2020 review: "There is low certainty evidence from nine trials (3507 participants) that wearing a mask may make little or no difference to the outcome of influenza-like illness (ILI) compared to not wearing a mask. ... There is moderate certainty evidence that wearing a mask probably makes little or no difference to the outcome of laboratory-confirmed influenza compared to not wearing a mask." [20] The language is purported to serve the interests of precision, but I've read enough of these to know that the language used here is more likely intended to blunt the hard fact that their research could not find substantive evidence supporting masks for use to control the spread of COVID-19.

The current political milieu restricts free expression of scientific opinion on matters related to COVID-19, more so in 2020 than it is at present. Perhaps that explains the contrast between the more recent, clear statement: "We are uncertain whether wearing masks or N95/P2 respirators helps to slow the spread of respiratory viruses based on the studies we assessed," and the earlier convoluted manner of expression: *"there is low certainty evidence ... that wearing a mask may make little or no difference."* In the latter, it's difficult to sort out what, exactly, the reviewer is saying. Is he saying evidence suggesting masks make little or no difference in the outcomes of influenza like sickness is of low certainty? So, there is evidence that masks make no difference, but it's of *low certainty*? Where is the evidence that they do provide at

---

//www.cochrane.org/CD006207/ARI_do-physical-measures-such-hand-washing-or-wearing-masks-stop-or-slow-down-spread-respiratory-viruses — 3/14/23] For PDF, see Doc Folder SE039

[20] Jefferson, Tom, Del Mar, Christ B., et al., *Physical interventions to interrupt or reduce the spread of respiratory viruses,* Cochrane Library, November 20, 2020 [ONLINE: https://www.cochranelibrary.com/cdsr/doi/10.1002/14651858.CD006207.pub5/full — 3/14/23] For PDF, see Doc. Folder SE039.02.

least some protection? Nothing is said about that. Clearly, the reviewers are admitting the evidence is on the side of *masks don't work* more than it is on the side of *masks work.*

The statement about *low certainty* regarding using masks to protect against influenza-like-illness (ILI) is followed by another convoluted statement, but less so, and we can gain insight from it to help us understand the first: *"there is moderate certainty evidence that wearing a mask probably makes little or no difference to the outcome of laboratory-confirmed influenza compared to not wearing a mask."* So, the evidence supporting the conclusion that masks make little or no difference in *laboratory-confirmed* cases is stronger than the evidence that masks provide *little or no* difference in the outcomes of influenza like sickness that is not confirmed by lab work.

I know! Getting a clear statement from these guys is sort of like trying to pick up mercury! And adding to the confusion, the Editor-in-Chief at Cochrane Library felt compelled to publish an explanation that their review was not intended to be taken as saying masks don't work.[21] But every intelligent person reading the review knows what it means. The Cochrane review is not talking about the certainty of evidence supporting masks, but rather making a comment on the evidence against masks. That's important! And it tells you that masks don't work "as advertised" by the medical establishment. Rather, they *work* as advertised on the boxes they come in: "Masks are not designed or intended to prevent, mitigate, treat, diagnose or cure any disease or health condition, including COVID-19/Coronavirus."[22]

---

[21] Soares-Weiser, Karla, Editor-in-Chief of the Cochrane Library, *Statement on 'Physical interventions to interrupt or reduce the spread of respiratory viruses' review,* Cochrane, March 10, 2023 [ONLINE: https://www.cochrane.org/news/statement-physical-interventions-interrupt-or-reduce-spread-respiratory-viruses-review.pdf — 3/14/23] For PDF, see Doc. Folder SE040.

[22] TEEPUBLIC, *Masks—Legal Disclaimer for Customers,* nd [ONLINE: https://teepublic.zendesk.com/hc/en-us/articles/360047284753-Masks-Legal-Disclaimer-for-Customers — 11/2/22] For PDF, see Doc. Folder OAI68.

The Bible warns us against *science falsely so called.* [23] This warning is an axiomatic affirmation of science *rightly so called.* So, by all means, let's follow true science.

____

[23] 1Timothy 6:20, "O Timothy, keep that which is committed to thy trust, avoiding profane and vain babblings, and oppositions of science falsely so called..." Fake science is no better than "vain babblings."

Chapter Two:
The research documentation used in this study, the thesis, and why I concentrated on studies that argue in support of mask use to control viral spread

Let's get right into the crux of this debate. 964 scientific research papers and articles were examined in preparation for this publication. More than half of these were articles specifically written or referenced to support mask use. Each of these was examined for any science proving the masks recommended by the medical establishment for our use during the pandemic provide protection from viral infection for the wearer or for the community. My notes, and a PDF of each article/study examined, are copied to my archives and available to anyone who is interested. All of this is available free with the purchase of this book. Contact me through www.godswar2020.com. I'll email the directions and coupon code. What follows is a summary of my findings.

What was I looking for in my research?

My Thesis Statement: The masks currently recommended for community use do not provide adequate protection from viral infection or contagion either as PPE (Personal Protective Equipment) or as source control (protecting the community from viral spread).

As a sub-thesis, I would add, the aforementioned masks do not pass a cost benefit analysis—there is greater harm than good in the equation.

I focused on research purporting to prove masks work

I concentrated on the articles gathered by one investigative reporter who asked, "Do face masks work?" He claimed to have assembled 49 "scientific studies that explain why they do." His name is Russell Falcon, and he reports for Austin, Texas NBC affiliate KXAN, as an In-Depth Investigative reporter. This article was published August 7, 2021, and updated December 23, 2021. Find it online at https://www.kxan.com/news/coronavirus/do-face-masks-work-here-are-49-scientific-studies-that-explain-why-they-do/ (as of June 25, 2021). I copied the article as a PDF (Portable Document Format) and it's available in my OR (Opposition Research) Doc. Folder as FN01.00.00.00.00. I refer to these articles collectively as the *Falcon articles, The Falcon* 49 or *Falcon's 49.* Of the 964 articles I examined in my research, 597 are connected with my examination of the *Falcon 49.*

I focused on the *Falcon articles* to fully acquaint myself with arguments supporting mask use to control the spread of a virus. It was important to discover if there was any study with scientific integrity that provided support for the masks recommended by the medical establishment and mandated by Federal government, some state and local governments, and some corporations.

Of the almost 600 studies I vetted in connection with *Falcon's 49*, only one was included that argued directly against the use of masks.[24] That article, together with the twelve articles referenced in it, was included because it came up in the course of my examination of the *Falcon articles*.

Not one article, not one RCT, not one observational study, or cohort, clinical, or controlled trial, or mathematical model, proved surgical or cloth masks provide adequate protection against viral infection.

I did not say none made that *claim.* Indeed, Falcon is correct to assert all the articles he named *claimed* mask efficacy, and many of them insinuated adequate efficacy to contribute significant protection against viral infection or contagion. But when these

---

[24] Center For Renewing America, staff, *POLICY BRIEF: COVID MASKS MANDATES PROVE BOTH INEFFECTIVE AND UNSUPPORTED BY THE EVIDENCE,* Center For Renewing America, September 17, 2021 [ONLINE: https://americarenewing. com/issues/policy-brief-covid-mask-mandates-prove-both-ineffective-and-unsupported-by-the-evidence/ — 11/17/22]. For PDF, see Doc. Folder SE01.00.00.00.00 and OR - FN01.43.01.00.00-FN01.43.03.00.00.

studies were examined by the criteria I established at the outset of my research, discussed in the pages of this book, not one survived the scrutiny.

In the following chapters, I will overview the science related to mask efficacy as PPE (Personal Protective Equipment—protection for the wearer) and then as source control (protection for the community by stopping the spread of viral droplets at the source). You will see that true science compels us to conclude *the masks recommended by Fauci and the government medical establishment do not provide adequate protection against a virus and so do not support their recommended use much less justify mask mandates.*

Chapter Three:
The ability of a mask to protect the wearer from viral infection

There is zero scientific support for the proposition that a surgical or cloth facemask will protect the wearer from viral infection. The following provides an overview of the evidence.

The Centers For Disease Control (CDC) affirms the consensus that mask filtering efficiency is a function of particle size.[25] SARS-CoV-2 particles are ~70-152 nm in diameter.[26] Surgical masks (SM) and cloth masks (CM) have pore sizes ranging from 300 nm

---

[25] Brosseau, Lisa, et. al. *N95 Respirators and Surgical Masks,* CDC, October 14, 2009 [ONLINE: https://blogs.cdc.gov/niosh-science-blog/2009/10/14/n95/ — 9/29/22] For PDF see Doc. Folder OR - FN01.38.00.03.29. "Further, the filter's collection efficiency is a function of the size of the particles, and is not dependent on whether they are bioaerosols or inert particles." See also Konda, Abhiteja, et. al., *Aerosol Filtration Efficiency of Common Fabrics Used in Respiratory Cloth Masks,* OSTI.GOV, US Department of Energy, Office of Scientific and Technical Information [ONLINE: https://www.osti.gov/biblio/1631577 — 9/29/22] For PDF see Doc. Folder OR - FN01.16.05.00.00. "Importantly, there is a need to evaluate filtration efficiencies as a function of aerosol particulate sizes in the 10 nm – 10 μm range, which is particularly relevant for respiratory virus transmission." [ONLINE: https://www.osti.gov/biblio/1631577-aerosol-filtration-efficiency-common-fabrics-used-respiratory-cloth-masks. FULL TEXT: https://www.osti.gov/servlets/purl/1631577.] For PDF, see Doc. Folder OR - FN01.16.05.00.00.

[26] Na Zhu, Ph.D., et al., *A Novel Coronavirus from Patients with Pneumonia in China*, New England Journal of Medicine, January 24, 2020 [ONLINE: https://www.nejm.org/doi/10.1056/NEJMoa2001017 — 9/25/22] For PDF, see Doc. Folder OR - FN01.37.01.02.00. The virus particle diameter measured from 60-140 nm. The spikes were measured at 9-12 nm, which, when added to the diameter rendered the full size range of the "corona" particles at 69-152 nm. The National Institute of Virology (ICMR) received a request for information regarding the size of SARS-CoV-2 particle, published October 11, 2021. [ONLINE https://awakenindiamovement. com/masks-pore-size/ — taken from www.Icmr.gov.in — 10/24/22] For PDF, see TECH71. "SARS-CoV-2 virus is round shaped with an average size of 70-80 nm."

(for the surgical masks) up to 500,000 nm (for the cloth masks).[27] (See footnote for scale of these sizes.)[28]

One study found *modified* surgical and cloth masks provided a percentage of filtration for particles in the 100 nm range. But the best performance was less than 80% capture, the materials used caused unacceptable breathing difficulties, and construction was complicated. [29] They are not recommended for public use.

Besides, the particle size range for SARS-CoV-2 is ~70-152 nm. [30] Only a very small portion of the hundreds of studies I examined tested masks for particles of this size. The NIOSH standard for testing mask efficacy is 300 nm and that is what virtually all studies followed. [31] According to OSHA, a properly

---

[27] You will find this stipulated in literature ubiquitously: the standard pore size of surgical masks ranges from 0.3-10 µm: see Awake India Movement publication of a formal request for information from ICMR-National Institute of Virology to the question "What is the pore size of the standard as well as surgical masks?" Answer: "Pore size of standard surgical mask and N95 mask is 0.3-10 µm & 0.1-0.3 µm respectively." [ONLINE: https://awakenindiamovement.com/masks-pore-size/ — 9/28/22]. For PDF, see Doc. Folder TECH71. For cloth masks (CM) see Bhanu Bhakta Neupane, et. al., *Optical microscopic study of surface morphology and filtering efficiency of face masks*, NIH, 2019 [ONLINE: https://www.ncbi.nlm.nih.gov/pmc/articles/PMC6599448/ — 9/29/22] For PDF, see Doc. Folder TECH70 or FN05: Speaking of CMs (cloth masks), authors said, "The pore size of masks ranged from 80 to 500 µm." That's 80,000 to 500,000 nanometers. SARS-2 virus particles, including the spikes, are roughly 70-150 nanometers in diameter.

[28] NOTE: To get some idea of scale when talking about micrometers (µm) and nanometers (nm) consider. A meter is roughly 3.5 feet. A millimeter (mm) is one one-thousandths of a meter. A micrometer (µm) is one one-thousandths of a millimeter (mm). A nanometer (nm) is one one-thousandths of a micrometer (µm). Beyond that we get into atomic sizes. I used the larger stipulated sizes for the SARS-2 virus, which includes the spike proteins that extend from the virion sphere creating its corona appearance.

[29] Clapp, Phillip, PhD, et. al., *Evaluation of Cloth Masks and Modified Procedure Masks as Personal Protective Equipment for the Public During the COVID-19 Pandemic*, JAMA Network, December 10, 2020 [ONLINE: https://jamanetwork.com/journals/jamainternalmedicine/article-abstract/2774266 — 9/29/22] For PDF, see Doc. Folder OR - FN01.16.00.00.00. For examination of this article, see *Let My People Breathe (Research Notes)*, p. 258

[30] IBID: Na Zhu, Ph.D., et al., *A Novel Coronavirus ...*

[31] NIOSH (National Institute for Occupational Safety and Health), published by CDC, effective date: April 8, 1998, [ONLINE: https://www.cdc.gov/niosh/npg/nengapdxe.html — 9/29/22] For PDF, see TECH74. "A high efficiency filter is at least 99.97% efficient against mono-disperesed [sic-dispersed] particles of 0.3 µm (micrometers) in diameter or higher." See also *42 CFR Part 84 Respiratory Protective Devices,* standards as of June 8, 1995, published by CDC [ONLINE: https://www.cdc.gov/niosh/npptl/topics/respirators/pt84abs2.html — 9/29/22] For PDF, see

fitted N95 blocks at least 95% of particles 300 nm in diameter.[32] No one recommends N95s for public use because they must be professionally fitted, cannot be worn for hours at a time because they are uncomfortable and restrict breathing, and should not be reused. That leaves the surgical or cloth masks. As pointed out earlier, the pore size of a standard surgical mask is 300 nm, and cloth mask pores range from 700 nm to 500,000 nm.[33] Do the math! A particle that is ~70-152 nanometers will very easily pass through a mask with pores that are ≥ 300 nm.[34] And this only accounts for penetration, that is, particles passing through the material of the mask; it doesn't take into consideration the problem of leakage, which allows particles to enter and escape through openings around the mask.[35]

Doc. Folder TECH77. "All filter tests will employ the most penetrating aerosol size, 0.3 μm aerodynamic mass median diameter."

[32] OSHA Review, *OSHA Requirements for Occupational Use of N95 Respirators in Healthcare,* OSHA, April 28, 2020 [ONLINE: https://oshareview.com/2020/04/osha-requirements-for-occupational-use-of-n95-respirators-in-healthcare/ — 9/29/22] For PDF, see TECH75. "When worn properly (with mask making a tight seal with the user's face), surgical N95 masks can filter at least 95% of very small (0.3 micron) test particles ..." 0.3 microns (μm) is equivalent to 300 nanometers (nm).

[33] IBID: You will find this stipulated in literature ubiquitously ...

[34] Shu-An Lee, et al., Respiratory Performance Offered by N95 Respirators and Surgical Masks: Human Subject Evaluation with NaCI Aerosol Representing Bacterial and Viral Range, Annals of Occupational Hygiene, Oxford University Press, 2008, [ONLINE: https://www.ncbi.nlm.nih.gov/pmc/articles/PMC7539566/#_ffn_sectitle — 11/17/22] For PDF, see Doc. Folder OR - FN01.38.00.03.35a. Go to DISCUSSION, toward the end of the second paragraph: "particles ... between 0.08 and 0.2 μm [80-200 nm] in aerodynamic diameter are more likely to penetrate into most of the tested N95 respirators. The respective size was 0.04-0.2 μm [40-200 nm] for surgical masks. Strikingly, the physical size of ... SARS-causing coronavirus is approximately 0.08-0.14 μm [80-140 nm], i.e. the size ranges of these viruses fall into the most penetrating particle size range." See also Wei Lyu, et al., Community Use of Face Masks And COVID-19: Evidence From A Natural Experiment Of State Mandates In The US, Health Affairs, VOL. 39, No. 8 [ONLINE: https://www.healthaffairs.org/doi/10.1377/hlthaff.2020.00818 — 2020; 9/24/22] For PDF, see Doc. Folder OR - FN01.40.00.00.00.

[35] Brosseau, LIsa, & Berry Ann, Roland, *N95 Respirators and Surgical Masks,* CDC, October14, 2009 [ONLINE: https://blogs.cdc.gov/niosh-science-blog/2009/10/14/n95/ — 9/28/22]. For PDF, see Doc. Folder OR - FN01.38.00.03.29. Authors stated two factors are critical for masks to be effective: "First, the filter must be able to capture the full range of sizes (<1 to >100 μm) .... Second, leakage must be prevented at the boundary of the facepiece and the face." See also Cumbo, Enzo et al., *Management and use of filter masks in the 'non-medical' population during the Covid-19 period,* ELSEVIER, Jan. 2021 [ONLINE: https://reader.elsevier.com/reader/sd/pii/S0925753520303945?token=2F4E086238A3BA6B3D

Surgical masks, properly fitted, and tested for direct attack penetration still do not perform at the threshold requirement of 80% efficiency at blocking particles that are ≤300 nm in diameter.[36] And when you talk about the typical cheap medical mask one buys at a local pharmacy, referred to as a *Barrier Face Covering* (BFC), it's even worse. These are not even rated by FDA or NIOSH, and they are known to be significantly inferior to a NIOSH approved surgical mask.[37]

By the way, *direct attack penetration* is when the particles are shot directly at the mask in a controlled environment. This is not a reasonable measure of surgical mask efficacy. Why? Masks for public use are nearly never fitted to seal off the open areas around the facemask. Doing so makes them virtually unbearable to wear all day. Loose fitting surgical masks leave openings around the nose, along the sides of the mouth, and often under the chin that allow for what is called *leakage*.[38] When honest researchers test surgical masks taking leakage into consideration, virtually all agree surgical or cloth masks are, practically speaking, worthless.[39] At

---

10AB873F63B75B14FB5E887DCDD2506B1661D41E7DD26A68A3513DA7E6979A712A731544F 5CED7&originRegion=us-east-1&originCreation=20220927204348 — 9/28/22]. For PDF, see Doc. Folder OR - FN01.41.06.00.00. Speaking of the problem of leakage: "Wearing a mask that does not adhere well to the face or even [sic] with the nose or mouth not covered properly, even makes the best device [mask, etc.] totally useless."

[36] IBID: *Clapp Phillip ...* Go to RESULTS and read along with my notes at p. 258ff in *Let My People Breathe (Research Notes).* For PDF, see Doc. Folder OR - FN01.16.00.00.00.

[37] Szalajda, Jonathan, et. al., *Overview of The ASTM F3502-21 Barrier Face Covering Standard,* CDC, April 23, 2021 [ONLINE: https://blogs.cdc.gov/niosh-science-blog/2021/04/23/bfc-standard/ — 9/29/22] For PDF, see Doc. Folder TECH81. The masks Fauci and company recommend for control of COVID-19 spread "don't have to meet federal standards to confirm their performance." According to this CDC published article, "ASTM (American Society for Testing and Materials) International, with input from NIOSH, recently developed a new Barrier Face Covering standard." They established two categories of filter efficiency (the number of particles captured by the mask): 20% and 50% — meaning the masks should meet a minimum standard of 20% filtration. It is absurd that any person of reason would think 20% or even 50% filtration is adequate to protect against transmission.

[38] IBID, Brosseau, Lisa, & Berry Ann, Roland, *N95 Respirators ...*

[39] IBID, Brosseau, Lisa, & Berry Ann, Roland, *N95 Respirators ...* NOTE: Keep in mind that when a researcher stipulates a size delimiter, such as ≤300 nm (meaning less than or equal to 300 nm), it does not mean to include every size below 300 nm. If the researcher could say the masks are effective to capture 20% of particles that are below, say, 200 nm, it is certain he or she would set

best, they rate at about 50% capture of particles that range from ≥500 nm to 5 μm (5,000 nm). Cloth masks are even worse. The pore size of a typical homemade cloth mask starts at about 700 nm.[40] Virions can blow through surgical and cloth facemasks like a mosquito through a chain-linked fence.

The Mosquito Through a Chain-Link Fence Analogy

One fellow responded to what he dubbed the "clever" mosquito analogy scoffing it's more like a mosquito riding a baseball through a chain link fence. This is because virus particles travel in droplets.

Okay, so the *baseball* is the droplet and the *mosquito* is the virus particle. I'll discuss the *droplet* issue in the next chapter. As we shall see, droplets evaporate almost instantly upon exposure to atmosphere, or via respiration and/or heat of the sun while sitting on the inside or outer surface of a mask. Furthermore, the droplets hit the mask at some velocity, and break down upon impact, quickly releasing the virion into the host or through the mask into the atmosphere. So, it's more like a mosquito riding a baseball that hits the chain link fence and sends the mosquito flying through. Or, it's like a mosquito riding a baseball made of water that breaks down upon contact with the fence and releases the mosquito to move on through. Or, it's like a mosquito trapped inside a liquid baseball that shrinks quickly, within milliseconds in most cases, before it even reaches the mask, releasing the mosquito ... you get the idea! So, whose' being clever now?

Not one RCT has supported any claim that masks protect against viral infection, and although the observational studies I examined varied widely, the standard surgical mask at best

---

the delimiter to ≤200 nm. For that reason, ≤300 nm virtually always bottoms out at 200+ nm. Remember that our criterion of concern involves particles that are from ~40-170 nm.

[40] Neupane, Bhanu Bhakta, et al., *Optical microscopic study of surface morphology and filtering efficiency of face masks,* March 21, 2019 [ONLINE: https://www.ncbi.nlm.nih.gov/pmc/articles/PMC6599448/ — 9/27/22] For PDF, see Doc. Folder OR - FN05. Examining the efficiency of cloth masks (CM), the authors wrote: "The pore size of masks ranged from 80 to 500 μm," which is 80,000 to 500,000 nanometers. The 700 nm is the lowest I found in any literature.

provided about 50%-70% for particles that were ≥300 nanometers making them wholly inadequate to protect the wearer from penetration of infectious virus particles.[41]

Wait! If the surgical mask captures up to 70% of the virions, doesn't that offer some real protection to the mask wearer?

No! First, keep in mind that I'm using the most generous estimates — in truth, when penetration and leakage are taken together, the average surgical masks hardly block above 25% of the particles. Nevertheless, taking the highest filtration estimates I found in all my research, 80% for a carefully fitted standard surgical mask, 20% penetration makes the mask meaningless.

It only takes one virion (infectious virus particle) to cause contagion. This is called the *Independent Action Hypothesis* (IAH). Since it is likely that thousands of particles assault a mask in the course of a day,[42] if the masks are allowing 20% of these through, they are providing zero benefit to the wearer. Think of it this way.

---

[41] Hyejung Jung, et al., Comparison of Filtration Efficiency and Pressure Drop in Anti-Yellow Sand Masks, Quarantine Masks, Medical Masks, General Masks, and Handkerchiefs, Taiwan Association for Aerosol Research, published in Aerosol and Air Quality Research, 2014 [ONLINE: https://aaqr.org/articles/aaqr-13-06-oa-0201.pdf — 9/28/22]. For PDF, see Doc. Folder OR - FN01.38.00.03.36. See Table 3 — According to Table 3, the surgical mask (SM) had an inward penetration of 59.083 rounded to 59% and outward penetration of 57.667, rounded to 58%. This means 59% of particles attacking the mask penetrated into the host, and 58% exhaled by the host penetrated the mask into atmosphere. Also, see my notes on this article: Let My People Breathe (Research Notes), p. 1168-1170.

[42] Stadnystkyi, Valentyn et. al., *The airborne lifetime of small speech droplets and their potential importance in SARS-CoV-2 transmission,* Proceedings of the National Academy of Science, USA, June 2020, published May 2020 [ONLINE: https://www.ncbi.nlm.nih.gov/pmc/articles/PMC7275719/#_ffn_sectitle — 9/28/22]. For PDF, see Doc. Folder OR - FN01.38.00.03.27. See *Let My People Breathe (Research Notes)*, pp. 1005-1016. You'll likely need my notes to sort out the numbers used in this article to quantify the volume of infectious particles in droplets. In Summary: Speaking produces thousands of oral droplets. 1 minute of loud speaking produces at least 1,000 droplets containing virions (infectious virus particles) in the form of droplet nuclei that remain airborne for more than 8 minutes. There can be 7 million strands of viral RNA in 1 mL of droplets (or 0.034 ounces). Bottom line: these researchers estimate 400 virions in each 5 μm droplet. The number of 5 μm droplets in one mL of ejecta is a possible staggering 600 trillion. If 37% of these contain infectious, or viral particles, you can see that there is a great deal of exposure assaulting the masks. Even if the mask blocked 80%, allowing only 20% penetration, it renders the masks worthless to protect against viral infection. But the truth is, the masks recommended by Fauci, et al., perform woefully below this threshold.

If you had a thousand bullets coming at your head, and you managed somehow to block 80% of those bullets, how many bullets engaging the target, your head, will it take to permanently eliminate your need to worry about COVID-19?

But in the case of virus particles penetrating a common surgical mask, the fact is it's more like 50%-75% are actually getting through.[43] So, it's a good thing we are not talking about bullets—the fact is COVID-19 has a survivability rate of above 98% across the board.[44] *Across the board* means this average includes the elderly and people with co-morbidities. Speaking of the elderly, those aged 75-79 survive COVID at a rate of 97%, and those over 80 at 92%.[45] When you narrow the focus to children, the death rate is virtually zero, with the age group 0-4 being slightly more vulnerable than the age group 5-14.[46] From 15-44 the survivability is virtually 100%.[47] 45-64 calculates out to 99.73% and 65-74 comes out to 98%.[48] Add morbidities at any age group, and survivability is significantly lower. But remember that these deaths are calculated into the survivability rates indicated above. It's also important to remember that multiple sources have revealed many

---

[43] Ueki, Hiroshi, et. al., *Effectiveness of Face Masks in Preventing Airborne Transmission of SARS-CoV-2,* American Society for Microbiology, September-October, 2020, published October 21, partially funded by NIAID [ONLINE: https://www.ncbi.nlm.nih.gov/pmc/articles/PMC7580955/#_ffn_sectitle — 9/29/22] For PDF, see Doc. Folder OR - FN01.36.01.06.00. Read my commentary on this article in *Let My People Breathe (Research Notes)*, pp. 634-649. Essentially, these researchers found surgical masks did not provide better than 50% filtration, which, of course, is totally inadequate to protect against viral infection.

[44] WebMD Medical Reference, Coronavirus Update: *Coronavirus Recovery,* reviewed by Melinda Tatini, DO, MS, January 25, 2022 [ONLINE: https://www.webmd.com/lung/covid-recovery-overview#3 — 9/28/22] For PDF, see Doc. Folder OAI41.

[45] Berezow, Alex, PhD, *COVID Infection Fatality Rates By Sex And Age,* published by American Council on Science and Health, Nov. 18, 2020. [ONLINE: https://www.acsh.org/news/2020/11/18/covid-infection-fatality-rates-sex-and-age-15163 — 9/28/22]. For PDF, see Doc. Folder OAI42.

[46] IBID: Berezow ... 0-4 0.003% (which looks like this: .00003) and 5-14 0.001% (or .00001).

[47] IBID: Berezow ... 15-19 through 40-44, adding the Mean dividing by 6 renders a death rate of 0.027% (or 99.973% survived)

[48] IBID: Berezow ...

reported COVID deaths are actually not attributable to COVID.[49] Because someone dies with COVID does not mean they died of that disease.

Nevertheless, even if the masks might capture some virus particles that doesn't mean they are providing to anyone protection from risk of contagion.

Epilogue on masks as protection for the wearer:

About mid to late 2021 researchers gave up on promoting the idea that the common surgical or cloth mask would provide any meaningful protection from viral infection, and they turned to arguing for *source control.*

The *white flag* was raised in surrender to the overwhelming evidence that surgical and cloth masks cannot provide adequate protection against particles that are smaller than 300 nm (most would stipulate to the limit being 500 nm). This is because even though most viral droplets begin at source in sizes large enough to be captured by a mask, they evaporate so quickly that by the time any reach by-standers, they are too small to be captured by a surgical or cloth mask.

Curiously, the general public was never made aware of this fact. And for over a year, the medical establishment, led by Fauci and friends, remained silent about it and allowed the people to believe the lie that masks could protect the wearer from a virus. Think about that! And understand it was not because they did not know better. There has never been a consensus in western science advocating for masks to be used for control of viral spread. People at Fauci's level knew this. Fauci agreed with that consensus, and said so in an email that we referenced earlier. Neither Fauci, nor

---

[49] Sacca, Paul, et al., *CDC's COVID Data Tracker revised COVID-19 deaths downward … ,* Health Feedback, March 24, 2022. More than 70,000 downward. [ONLINE: https://healthfeedback.org/claimreview/cdcs-covid-data-tracker-deaths-downward-reliable-data-still-indicate-covid-19-major-cause-of-death/ — 9/28/22] For PDF, see Doc. Folder OAI43. This is one of many examples that could be cited, but since it amounts to a mea culpa by the CDC, I reckoned it sufficient to support the point.

any medical *leaders* in the US presented us with any scientific study that proved otherwise. The fact is, these people lied to us!

When the truth proved stubborn and refused to surrender to this absurd lie, the government medical establishment relented and everyone shifted to a focus on source control (capturing particles at the source).

Masks do not protect the wearer from contagion by a virus. But, what about source control? Can masks provide protection for the community?

Chapter Four:
The shift from masks as protection for the wearer to masks as protection for the community:

Source control refers to stopping the spread of virus at the *source,* and involves capturing the particles before they are exhaled into the atmosphere when people breathe, talk, sing, shout, cough, or sneeze.

Particles are carried in droplets that begin at source much larger than the *naked virus* (from 5-10 μm, or 5000-10000 nm,[50] verses the naked virus which is ~70-152 nm).[51] Surgical and some

---

[50] Droplet sizes are classified in different ways; what follows is a brief summary: CDC classifies "fine particles" as any <10 μm: *Science Brief: Community Use of Masks to Control the Spread of SARS-CoV-2,* December 6, 2021 [ONLINE: https://www.cdc.gov/coronavirus/2019-ncov/science/science-briefs/masking-science-sars-cov2.html?CDC_AA_refVal=https%3A%2F%2Fwww.cdc.gov%2Fcoronavirus%2F2019-ncov%2Fmore%2Fmasking-science-sars-cov2.html — 11/17/22] For PDF, see Doc. Folder OR - FN01.36.01.00.00 & FN01.39.02.00.00. Industrial hygienists categorize droplets according to how deeply they penetrate the respiratory system: respirable aerosols — into the lungs (<2.5 μm, noted as PM2.5 (*Particulate Matter* followed by size in micrometers)); thoracic aerosols — into the trachea (<10 to 15 μm, PM10); inhalable aerosols — into nose and throat (100-200 μm, PM100): see Milton, *A Rosetta Stone for Understanding Infectious Drops and Aerosols,* Journal of the Pediatric Infectious Disease Society, Oxford U Press, July, 2020 [ONLINE: https://www.ncbi.nlm.nih.gov/pmc/articles/PMC7495905/ — 11/107/22] For PDF, see Doc. Folder OR - FN01.38.00.03.28. Droplets that remain airborne indefinitely are called aerosols. The consensus, until lately, has been any particle <5μm is an aerosol: Lowen, et. al., *Influenza virus transmission is dependent on relative humidity and temperature*, Public Library of Science Pathogens (PLoS Pathog,) 2007 [ONLINE: https://www.ncbi.nlm.nih.gov/pmc/articles/PMC2034399/] For PDF, see Doc. Folder OR - FN01.38.00.03.35b. Howard, Jeremy et al., *An evidence review of face masks against COVID-19,* Proceedings of the National Academy of Science, January 26, 2021 [ONLINE: https://www.ncbi.nlm.nih.gov/pmc/articles/PMC7848583/#_ffn_sectitle — 10/2/22] For PDF, see Doc. Folder OR - FN01.38.00.03.03. "The smallest particles (≤5 μm) able to reach into the respiratory bronchioles and alveoli in the lungs and medium-sized ones (up to 10 μm to 15 μm) able to deposit in 'the trachea and large intrathoracic airways'." Before COVID, the cut off was 5μm: "Coarse" sized particles were regarded as those >5 μm and "fine" sized particles were set at ≤5 μm, see Milton, Donald et al., *Influenza Virus Aerosols in Human Exhaled Breath: Particle Size, Culturability, and Effect of Surgical Masks,* PLoS Pathog., March 9, 2013 [ONLINE: https://www.ncbi.nlm.nih.gov/pmc/articles/PMC3591312/#_ffn_sectitle — 10/2/22] For PDF, see Doc. Folder OR - FN01.38.00.14.00.

[51] IBID: Na Zhu, Ph.D., et al., *A Novel Coronavirus ...*

cloth masks can capture droplets ≥5 μm (5000 nm).[52] Leaders in the medical establishment, who advocated for these masks as personal protection, finally conceded to the science, and maneuvered to a fallback position: the debate shifted from the ability of surgical masks to capture particles in droplets ≤ 300 nm to their ability to capture virus droplets at source, when they are much larger.

Since all attention was turned to masks as *source control*, I shifted the focus of my research to another question: *Do masks provide effective protection for the community?*

Overview of essential facts:

Ejecta refer to the material *ejected* from the body via exhaling during natural respiration, talking, coughing, or sneezing.

From the source (the person breathing, talking, sneezing, or coughing) droplets are expressed into ambient air as a cloud, or a plume in a wide variety of sizes. [53] This plume includes more material than only the virus particles, such as bacteria, and fungi spores.[54]

A *virus droplet* is a bead of moisture that contains at least one virus particle, but can include many. Most of the droplets exhaled

---

[52] Milton, Donald K. et al., *Influenza Virus Aerosols in Human Exhaled Breath: Particle Size, Culturability, and Effect of Surgical Masks,* Public Library of Science Pathogens (PLoS Pathog.), March 9, 2013 [ONLINE: https://www.ncbi.nlm.nih.gov/pmc/articles/ PMC3591312/#_ffn_sectitle — 10/2/22] For PDF, see Doc. Folder OR - FN01.38.00.14.00. After testing surgical masks for efficacy to capture particles in a range of 0.05-50 μm (50-50,000 nm), Milton, et al. concluded with an earlier study referred to as *Johnson, et al.* as follows: "We view results from Johnson et al and the present study as complementary. Together the studies show that surgical masks can limit the emission of large droplet spray and aerosol droplets larger than 5 μm [16]. However, surgical masks are not as efficient at preventing release of very small particles. It is well known that surgical masks are not effective for preventing exposure to fine particles when worn as personal protection.[18]"

[53] IBID: Valentyn Stadnystkyi, et. al.,

[54] Cedars-Sinai Staff, *Viruses, Bacteria and Fungi: What's the Difference?* Cedars-Sinai, June 17, 2020 [ONLINE: https://www.cedars-sinai.org/blog/germs-viruses-bacteria-fungi.html — 10/17/22] For PDF, see Doc. Folder TECH87, and Carpagnano, et al., *Analysis of the fungal microbiome in exhaled breath condensate of patients with asthma,* PubMed.gov, May 2016 [ONLINE: https://pubmed.ncbi.nlm.nih.gov/27178886/ — 10/17/22] For PDF, see Doc. Folder TECH88.

do not contain infectious virus particles.[55] Nevertheless, infectious virus RNA is found in exhaled breath even from normal respiration.[56]

Larger droplets fall to the surface quickly (>500 μm in under one second—0.6 s),[57] but many remain airborne for a significant amount of time and those <5 μm (5000 nm) can remain airborne indefinitely as aerosols.[58] An aerosol is a droplet that is free-

---

[55] Leung, et al., *Respiratory virus shedding in exhaled breath and efficacy of face masks*, Nature Medicine, April, 2020 [ONLINE: https://www.ncbi.nlm.nih.gov/pmc/articles/PMC8238571/ — 11/17/22] For PDF, see Doc. Folder OR - FN01.28.03.00.00. "Among the samples collected without a face mask, we found that the majority of participants with influenza virus and coronavirus infection did not shed detectable virus in respiratory droplets or aerosols." See also Eikenberry, Steffen et al., *To mask or not to mask: Modeling the potential for face mask use by the general public to curtail the COVID-19 pandemic,* KeAI Publishing, April 6, 2020 [ONLINE: https://www.ncbi.nlm.nih.gov/pmc/articles/PMC7186508/ — 11/17/22] For PDF, see Doc. Folder OR - FN01.41.07.00.00.

[56] Fabian, Patricia et al., *Influenza Virus in Human Exhaled Breath: An Observational Study*, PLOS ONE, July 2008 [ONLINE: https://www.ncbi.nlm.nih.gov/pmc/articles/PMC2442192/?report=reader] For PDF, see Doc. Folder OR - FN01.41.08.02.05. "In the present study, we measured generation rates of <192 and 1200 influenza virus RNA copies per hour for subjects with detectable influenza virus RNA in their breath." See also Anfinrud, Philip et al., *Could SARS-CoV-2 be transmitted via speech droplets?* MedRxiv, April 6, 2020 [ONLINE: https://www.medrxiv.org/content/10.1101/2020.04.02.20051177v1.full.pdf — 11/17/22] For PDF, see Doc. Folder OR - FN01.38.00.03.39b. Experiment showed ~900 droplets of varying sizes were produced in a 20 second time frame by subject repeating "Stay Healthy." In a fifteen-minute period, one person could emit over 40,000 droplets during normal speaking.

[57] Anchordoqui, Luis A. & Chudnovsky, Eugene M. (physicists) *A Physicist View of COVID-19 Airborne Infection through Convective Airflow in Indoor Spaces,* SciMedicine Journal, Received August 2, 2020, Accepted August 25, 2020 [ONLINE: https://www.researchgate.net/publication/343946982_A_Physicist_View_of_COVID-19_Airborne_Infection_through_Convective_Airflow_in_Indoor_Spaces/download — 10/13/22] For PDF, see Doc. Folder TECH86. See p. 69, examines settling (sedimenting) rates versus evaporation. Droplets settle as follows: Droplet size / Settling time: >500 μm / 0.6 s (seconds); ~50 μm / 6 s; ~5 μm / 600 s (~10 minutes); ~0.5 μm / 60,000 s, ~ 16.6 hrs).

[58] Siddhartha, Verma et al. *Visualizing the effectiveness of face masks in obstructing respiratory jets,* PMC, AIP Publishing, June 2020 [ONLINE: www.ncbi.nlm.nih.gov/pmc/articles/PMC7327717/ — 10/12/22]. For PDF, see Doc. Folder OR - FN01.36.01.04.00. "The smallest droplets and particles (diameter <5 μm-10 μm) may remain suspended in the air indefinitely..." A NIAID (Fauci) partially funded study by Hiroshi, et al., *Effectiveness of Face Masks in Preventing Airborne Transmission of SARS-CoV-2,* NCBI, NIH, Oct. 2020 defined aerosols as including particles that are 5.5 μm in diameter. [ONLINE: www.ncbi.nlm.nih.gov/pmc/articles/ PMC7580955/ — 10/12/22] For PDF, see Doc. Folder OR - FN01.36.01.06.00.

floating and carried about by air currents. These are usually ≤5 μm (5000 nanometers).

Visible droplets (~55-75 μm and larger)[59] begin evaporating immediately. A 50 μm (50,000 nm) droplet reaches full desiccation in less than 1 second (0.4 s), and a 100 μm droplet in under 2 (1.7 s).[60] When droplets reach full desiccation, they become what are called *droplet-nuclei*, which are described as "a dried-out spherical mass consisting of the particulate contents."[61] These droplet-nuclei are smaller than 10 μm, inhalable, and potentially infectious.[62] They quickly become aerosolized particles that can free float indefinitely as they continue to shrink due to evaporation. Within milliseconds, in most conditions, and in only a few seconds at most in virtually all other environments, droplets release virions (infectious particles) that are from 0.07-0.2 μm (70-200 nm), which are too small to be captured by the recommended masks. Remember that the most penetrating particle size for an N95 is

---

[59] Short-Fact Admin, *What is the smallest size visible to the naked eye?* Short-Fact, April 2021 [ONLINE: https://short-fact.com/what-is-the-smallest-size-visible-to-the-naked-eye/ — 10/12/22]. For PDF, see Doc. Folder TECH85. Particle size classification varies broadly. Lydia Bourouiba, PhD., observed the "classification systems employ various arbitrary droplet diameter cutoffs, from 5 to 10 μm" — cutoff refers to the dichotomy between *large* and *small* droplet categories: Bourouiba, Lydia, PhD., *Turbulent gas clouds and respiratory pathogens* ... JAMA Insights, March 26, 2020. [ONLINE: https://jamanetwork.com/journals/jama/fullarticle/2763852 — 10/13/22]. For PDF, see Doc. Folder OR - FN01.41.05.01.00. Bourouiba also notes that droplets do not evaporate uniformly: droplets in a cloud, or plume, desiccate more slowly than when isolated. The range is from milliseconds to minutes.

[60] IBID. Anchordoqui, Luis A., *A Physicist View of COVID-19 Airborne Infection through Convective Airflow in Indoor Spaces,* SciMedicine Journal, vol. 2, Special Issue "COVID-19", August 2, 2020 [ONLINE: https-//www.researchgate.net/publication/ 343946982 _A_Physicist_View_of_COVID-19_Airborne_Infection_through_Convective_Airflow_in_Indoor_Spaces/download — 10/13/22] For PDF, see Doc. Folder TECH86. EVAPORATION: a 50 μm droplet will reach desiccation (complete evaporation) in 0.4 seconds. See Table 1. Evaporation Time of Water Droplets, p. 70.

[61] Nicas, Mark et al., *Toward understanding the risk of secondary airborne infection: Emission of respirable pathogens,* Journal of Occupational Environmental Hygiene, 2005 [ONLINE: https://www.ncbi.nlm.nih.gov/pmc/articles/PMC7196697/ — 10/13/22] For PDF, see Doc. Folder OR - FN01.36.01.04.01.

[62] Loeb, Mark et. al., *Surgical Mask vs N95 Respirator,* JAMA Network, 2009 [ONLINE: https://jamanetwork.com/ journals/jama/fullarticle/184819 — 10/13/22] For PDF, see Doc. Folder OR - FN01.38.00.08.01. These droplet nuclei can be infectious: "inhalational transmission with small droplet nuclei (<10 μm) can occur."

from 0.1 to 0.3 microns (μm), or 100-300 nm.[63] For FDA cleared surgical masks it's 200-500 nm.[64]

The invisible droplets range from 10 μm (10,000 nanometers) down into *nano* sized droplets <1 μm. It is generally agreed that most of the droplets from source are from 5μm-10μm. These droplets fall much more slowly, and in certain conditions evaporate almost immediately into aerosols.

"Source control devices...collect respiratory particles larger than 0.3 μm primarily by impaction."[65] Droplets impact the mask at some velocity[66] and begin breaking down immediately,[67] which facilitates evaporation.[68]

---

[63] Qian, Willeke, Grinshpun & Donnelly, *Performance of N95 Respirators: Filtration Efficiency for Airborne Microbial and Inert Particles,* PubMed via ResearchGate, March 1998 [ONLINE: Abstract only: https://www.researchgate.net/publication/13743342_ Performance_of_N95_Respirators_Filtration_Efficiency_for_Airborne_Microbial_and_Inert_Particles — 10/17/22] For PDF, see Doc. Folder OR - FN01.38.00.03.38b2. Note: this is for N95s.

[64] Rengasamuy, Samy et al., *Filtration Performance of FDA-Cleared Surgical Masks,* Journal of the International Society for Respiratory Protection, July 13, 2020 [ONLINE: https://www.ncbi.nlm.nih.gov/pmc/articles/PMC7357397/#_ffn_sectitle — 10/17/22] For PDF, see Doc. Folder OR - FN01.16.01.00.00. "Surgical masks showed penetration levels of approximately 55-85% and 70-90% at flow rates of 30 and 100 liters/minute, respectively, for 300 nm particles. The most penetrating particle size (MPPS) was in the 200-500 nm range."

[65] Lindsley, William G. et al. *Efficacy of face masks, neck gaiters and face shields for reducing the expulsion of simulated cough-generated aerosols,* CDC & NIOSH, November 2020 [ONLINE: https://www.tandfonline.com/doi/full/10.1080/02786826. 2020.1862409 — 10/17/22] For PDF, see Doc. Folder OR - FN01.39.02.00.00.

[66] For an intriguing study of this phenomenon, see Bergeron & Quere, *Water droplets make an impact,* physicsworld, May, 2001 [ONLINE: https://physicsworld.com/a/water-droplets-make-an-impact/ — 10/17/22] For PDF, see Doc. Folder TECH89. See also Dbouk, Talib & Drikakis, Dimitris, *On respiratory droplets and face masks,* AIP Publishing: Physics of Fluids, May 23, 2020, published June 16, 2020 [ONLINE: https://aip.scitation.org/doi/10.1063/5.0015044#suppl — 11/17/22] For PDF, see Doc. Folder OR - FN01.38.00.03.35.

[67] Melayil & Mitra, *Wetting, Adhesion, and Droplet Impact on Face Masks,* Langmuir, American Chemical Society, March 2, 2021 [ONLINE: https://www.ncbi.nlm.nih.gov/pmc/articles/PMC7901139/#_ffn_sectitle — 10/17/22] For PDF, see Doc. Folder OR - FN01.38.00.34c.

[68] IBID. Anchordoqui, Luis A. & Chudnovsky, Eugene M. For PDF, see Doc. Folder TECH86. See p. 70, examines evaporation times noting that the smaller droplets desiccate more quickly: Droplet Diameter in μm / Evaporation Time in seconds: 2000 / 660 s; 1000 / 165 s; 500 / 41 s; 200 / 6.6 s; 100 / 1.7 s; 50 / 0.4 s. For a close examination of droplet evaporation on porous and nonporous materials see Goncalves, et al., *Droplet evaporation on porous fabric materials,* Scientific Reports, January 20, 2022 [ONLINE: https://www.nature.com/articles/s41598-022-04877-w — 10/18/22]

So, what does this mean?

Application of the facts:

As I poured over my research, I painstakingly sought for any scientific evidence supporting the idea that masks provide protection for the larger community, even if they don't provide protection for the wearer. From the research outlined above, and what follows, here is what I discovered.

1. Not all virus particles begin as droplets that are ≥ 5000 nm; a significant number of much smaller particles are emitted during normal talking, which can escape through the recommended masks.[69] These present all the challenges of virus penetrating through mask materials that we have discussed earlier.

2. Many larger and smaller particles escape capture by the masks through leakage[70] (around openings created by masks not sealed to the face).[71]

For PDF, see Doc. Folder TECH91. In summary, droplets begin imbibition (absorption) immediately upon contact with porous material and spread, which enhances evaporation. On nonporous material, the evaporation time is extended. But in every case, reduction in droplet mass continues and depending on factors like humidity and exposure to air movement desiccates over a very short time, exposing source and public to released droplet nuclei.

[69] Netz, Roland R., & Eaton, William A., *Physics of virus transmission by speaking droplets,* Biological Sciences, Brief Report, September 24, 2020 [ONLINE: https://www.pnas.org/doi/10.1073/pnas.2011889117 — 10/17/22] For PDF, see Doc. Folder TECH92. "Can we say anything useful about the number of emitted virions while speaking? Table 1 shows the calculated values for initial droplet radii ... from 1 μm to 40 μm ... predicts that the number of emitted virions per minute of continuously speaking ranges from 3 to ~2 x 10^5," or, 3 to about 2 million virions. See also Stadnytskyi, et al., *The airborne lifetime of small speech droplets and their potential importance in SARS-CoV-2 transmission,* Biological Sciences, Brief Report, May 13, 2020 [ONLINE: https://www.pnas.org/doi/10.1073/pnas.2006874117 — 10/18/22] For PDF, see Doc. Folder OR - FN01.38.00.03.27 (The NIH.gov published article). "It is less widely known that normal speaking also produces thousands of oral fluid droplets with a broad size distribution (*ca.* 1 μm to 500 μm)."

[70] Dbouk, Talib, & Drikakis, Dimitris, *On respiratory droplets and face masks,* Physics of Fluids, AIP Publishing, June 1, 2020 [ONLINE: https://www.ncbi.nlm.nih.gov/pmc/articles/PMC7301882/#__ffn_sectitle — 10/18/22] For PDF, see Doc. Folder OR - FN01.38.00.03.34b.

[71] Weber, Angela et al., *Aerosol penetration and leakage characteristics of masks used in the health care industry,* AJIC (American Journal of Infection Control), Vol. 21, Number 4, August 1993 [ONLINE: https://www.ajicjournal.org/article/0196-6553(93)90027-2/pdf — 10/18/22]. For

Certain mechanisms of physics and aerodynamics actually jet particles through leakage with even greater force than would occur without a mask.

3.   Droplets large enough to be trapped inside a mask begin desiccation (evaporation) immediately, which is facilitated, or sped up, by respiration.[72] Soon, every droplet evaporates, releasing the virion to be exhaled into aerosol, or allowing it to be inhaled with great force deep into the lower respiratory tract where there is the greatest risk for infection.[73] In other words, even those droplets trapped at source will not stop the decomposition of the droplet, and eventual evaporation, allowing the virions to escape.

4.   Droplet moisture gathering on the inside of a common surgical or cloth mask is not only uncomfortable, but can also increase restricted airflow, and exacerbate problems long associated with prolonged use of masks. Acne, follicle occlusion causing lumps, or nodules that can become inflamed and painful, changes in the skin microflora around the masked area which can cause rashes, hypoxia (reduced oxygen levels in the blood) and dyspnea (shortness of breath during exertion), to name a few of the problems associated with prolonged face mask use.[74] Masks were

---

PDF, see Doc. Folder OR - FN01.38.00.03.38b. "Filter penetration ranged from 20% to nearly 100% for submicrometer sized particles. ... When the surgical masks had artificially induced face-seal leaks, the concentration of submicrometer sized particles inside the mask increased slightly ... We conclude the protection provided by surgical masks may be insufficient ..."

[72] IBID. Anchordoqui, Luis A. & Chudnovsky, Eugene M. For PDF, see Doc. Folder TECH86

[73] Zhao, Mervin et al., *Household Materials Selection for Homemade Cloth Face Coverings and Their Filtration Efficiency Enhancement with Triboelectric Charging*, American Chemical Society, Nano Letters, June 2, 2020 [ONLINE: https://www.ncbi.nlm.nih.gov/pmc/articles/PMC7294826/#_ffn_sectitle — 10/18/22] For PDF, see Doc. Folder OR - FN01.38.00.03.38. "Larger particles >5 µm in diameter typically settle due to gravity and usually reach only the upper respiratory tract if inhaled. Meanwhile, fine particles with diameter <5 µm can critically reach the lower respiratory tract."

[74] Purushothaman, P. K., Priyangha, E., and Vaidhyswaran, Roopak, *Effects of Prolonged Use of Facemasks on Healthcare Workers in Tertiary Care Hospital During COVID-19 Pandemic*, Indian Journal of Otolaryngology and Head & Neck Surgery, March 2021 [ONLINE: https://www.ncbi.nlm.nih.gov/pmc/articles/PMC7490318/#_ffn_sectitle — 10/20/22] For PDF, see Doc. Folder OAI45. Nguyen, Jennifer & Nixon, Rosemary (Dermatologists), *Skin reactions to face*

never meant to be worn for hours at a time. Hypoxia, even at low levels, depresses the immune system by inhibiting the type of immune cells the body uses to fight viral infections.[75]

5.   No masks block a sufficient number of droplets from 300 nm to 500 nm so as to insure protection against infection, since at best, they only provide 20-50% filtration at that size, meaning 80-50% escape capture.[76] In the extreme scenario, say only 10-20% of the expressed virions escape capture, according to the rule of IAH (Independent Action Hypothesis) any one particle can cause

---

masks, DermNet, April, 2021 [ONLINE: https://dermnetnz.org/topics/skin-reactions-to-face-masks — 10/20/22] For PDF, see Doc. Folder OAI46

[75] Blaylock, Russell, *Blaylock: Face Masks Pose Serious Risks To The Healthy,* TECHNOCRACY, October 19, 2022 [ONLINE: https://www.technocracy.news/blaylock-face-masks-pose-serious-risks-to-the-healthy/.pdf — 10/20/22]. For PDF, see Doc. Folder OAI44. "Dr. Russell Blaylock warns that not only do face masks fail to protect the healthy from getting sick, but they also create serious health risks to the wearer." A "study of surgical masks found significant reductions in blood oxygen ..." And "the longer the duration of wearing the [surgical] mask, the greater the fall in blood oxygen levels." "The importance of these findings is that a drop in oxygen levels (hypoxia) is associated with an impairment in immunity."

[76] Droegemeier, Kevin, PhD, *Rapid Expert Consultation Update on SARS-CoV-2 Surface Stability and Incubation for the COVID-19 Pandemic,* Office of Science and Technology Policy, March 27, 2020 [ONLINE: https://www.ncbi.nlm.nih.gov/books/ NBK556956/?report=reader — 10/20/22] For PDF, see Doc. Folder OR - FN01.38.00.03.39a. "A mask made from a four-layer woven handkerchief ... had a 0.7% filtration efficiency for 0.3 micron size particles... Much higher filtration efficiency was observed with filters created specifically for the research from a five-layer woven brushed fabric (35.3% of the particles were trapped) and from four layers of polyester knitted cut-pile fabric (50% of the particles were trapped..." Note that the challenge was for particles 300 nm, and included masks that were specially made, the sort you cannot purchase in a store. For more documentation supporting the claim that the best surgical and cloth masks can do is fairly represented as about 50% filtration, see the following: Zhao, Mervin, et al., *Household Materials Selection for Homemade Cloth Face Coverings and Their Filtration Efficiency Enhancement with Triboelectric Charging,* American Chemical Society, Nano Letters, June 2, 2020 [ONLINE: https://www.ncbi.nlm.nih.gov/pmc/articles/ PMC7294826/#_ffn_sectitle — 10/20/22] For PDF, see Doc. Folder OR - FN01.38.00.03.38. The best performing cotton filters provided 20-26% filtration (see Table 2, where electrostatic charged polypropylene masks (PP-4) provided only 10-20% filtration. In the particle size range of 78-95 nm, the best performance masks allowed 50-60% penetration: Howard, Jeremy et al., *An evidence review of face masks against COVID-19,* January 26, 2021 [ONLINE: https://www.ncbi.nlm.nih.gov/pmc/ articles/PMC7848583/#_ffn_sectitle — 10/20/22] For PDF, see Doc. Folder OR - FN01.38.00.03.00. One more: Ueki, Hiroshi et al., *Effectiveness of Face Masks in Preventing Airborne Transmission of SARS-CoV-2,* American Society For Microbiology, mSphere, October 21, 2020 [ONLINE: https://www.ncbi.nlm.nih.gov/pmc/articles/PMC7580955/#_ffn_sectitle — 10/20/22] For PDF, see Doc. Folder OR - FN01.36.01.06.00. The best these researchers could get from a surgical mask is 50% filtration of particles > 1 μm.

infection. Consider this in view of the scientific proof that multiple thousands of particles are generated in 15 to 30 minutes speech, one cough, or sneeze, etc. In the course of a day, multiple thousands of virions escape from the mask. If only 10% or 20% escape capture, the chances for infection are such that make the mask worthless. Remember the bullet analogy used earlier? How many virions landing on target does it take to make the mask meaningless? (Happily, the risk of infection is not as high, and the risk of death from the disease caused by the SARS-CoV-2 virus is much lower than we have been led to believe.)

6. Finally, to support the claim that surgical masks have a capture rate of 85-98% for particles that are ≥5 μm, they must ignore leakage, and disregard the fact that smaller particles do escape capture at source. I found it intriguing that consensus formed around the claim that surgical masks, the type recommended by Fauci, et al., efficiently capture droplets that are ≥5 μm. [77] Interestingly, it turns out that our natural filtration system is very efficient at capturing particles in this size range, and does a far superior job.

This takes us to the most exciting part of our examination of the science: natural filtration!

---

[77] When one examines my research of the *Falcon 49* organized chronologically (See Doc. Folder OR Research — CHRONOLOGICAL TABLE), western pre-COVID researchers consistently defined aerosols as smaller than 5 μm, and the question was whether masks protected against submicron sized virus particles (<1 μm), including submicron sized microdroplets. Post COVID, this began to change. The "science" slowly redefined the criteria for classification of aerosols to include droplets that were from 5 μm to 10 μm. This allowed medical researchers to claim masks effectively captured "aerosols." Almost all the testing involved attacking the fabric of the masks directly, which virtually assumed perfect sealing and thus ignored leakage altogether. In other words, a chronological ordering of my extensive research shows a clear pattern exposing what appears to be a purposed effort to manipulate special definitions in order to support the mask mandate narratives.

Chapter Five:
Natural Filtration Versus Masks

The recommended masks interfere with our natural filtration system, and in fact aid and abet the virus attack.

We are told to follow the science. That's what I did! It led me to the conclusion that masks are ineffective either as PPE or CPE (source control via *community protective equipment*).

But I stumbled upon something that was amazing! God's natural filtration system is much more effective than masks.

Our nose and nasal cavity captures particles in the ≥ 5 µm size range,[78] and coats them with mucous.[79] About 60% of particles "smaller than 3 µm and larger than 0.5 µm are filtered by the nasal mucosa and transported by cilia propulsion to the nasopharynx."[80]

---

[78] Druguid, J. P., *THE SIZE AND THE DURATION OF AIR-CARRIAGE OF RESPIRATORY DROPLETS AND DROPLET-NUCLEI,* The Department of Bacteriology, Edinburgh University, 1946 [ONLINE: https://www.ncbi.nlm.nih.gov/pmc/articles/PMC2234804/pdf/jhyg00188-0053.pdf — 10/29/22] For PDF, see Doc. Folder OR - FN01.38.00.20.01. "The size of the droplet nuclei is of further importance, for it determines the part of the respiratory tract on to which the nuclei will be deposited when they are inhaled. According to Hatch (1942), most particles larger than 5 µ [equivalent to current notation µm] in diameter are deposited by centrifugal force in the upper respiratory tract (nasal cavity), while many particles smaller than 5 µ are deposited by settlement in the alveoli of the lungs ..." A more current study corroborates Druguid and adds further insight: Dhnad, Rajiv & Li, Jie, *Coughs and Sneezes: Their Role in Transmission of Respiratory Viral Infections, Including SARS-CoV-2,* American Journal of Respiratory and Critical Care Medicine, American Thoracic Society, June 16, 2020 [ONLINE: https://www.ncbi.nlm.nih.gov/pmc/articles/PMC7462404/ #_ffn_sectitle — 10/29/22] For PDF, see Doc. Folder OAI51. "Particles >5 µm in aerodynamic diameter are most likely to deposit by impaction in the oropharynx and be swallowed." NOTE: Particles <5 µm can bypass impaction and enter into the lungs. Those even smaller can move through the bronchial passages and enter the alveoli, where they can pass into the blood.

[79] Sanchez, Edith, *What Is Nasal Mucus and What Does It Do?* SteptoHealth, May 26, 2022 [ONLINE: https://steptohealth.com/ what-is-nasal-mucus-and-what-does-it-do/ — 10/29/22] For PDF, see Doc. Folder OAI50. "Nasal mucus ... main function has to do with preventing unwanted particles from entering the respiratory system." Helps "trap and expel foreign particles that enter the nose. ... this includes dust, pollen, bacteria and viruses."

[80] Schwab, Jan-Alexander MD & Zenkel, Matthias MD, *Filtration of Particulates in the Human Nose,* Wiley Online Library: The Laryngoscope, January 1998 [ONLINE:

The nasopharynx contains adenoid tissue, which serves as part of the immune system, attacking foreign particles with white blood cells to ward off infection. [81] Material accumulating in the nasopharynx cavity "drains into the throat, nose or ears."[82] From the throat it is swallowed where virions are neutralized in gastric acids; from the nose it is discharged through blowing ones nose or sneezing. If the body identifies particles trapped in the nasal passageway as potentially infectious, histamine triggers a production of more mucus, immune cells begin attacking the unwanted particles, and the build up of mucus agitates the host to clear his or her nose, ejecting the foreign particles by blowing the nose or by sneezing.[83] Proper hygiene is all that is necessary to capture and discard the ejecta in a sanitary fashion.

Particles >5 µm drawn in through the mouth are usually caught by impaction against the oropharynx and swallowed into the gastric chamber where they are neutralized,[84] or ejected through coughing. [85] Ordinary coughing etiquette is sufficient to discharge these virions safely. (Keep in mind, that coughing into a mask provides virtually no protection to the wearer or community, as we have previously shown.)

Filtration of particles "smaller than 0.5 µm [<500 nanometers] is low. They seem to pass easily into the lower respiratory tract."[86]

---

https://onlinelibrary.wiley.com/doi/full/10.1097/00005537-199801000-00023 — 11/1/22] For PDF, see Doc. Folder OAI52.

[81]Healthline Editorial Team, *Nasopharynx,* healthline/Human Body/Respiratory System/Nasopharynx, May 30, 2018 [ONLINE: https://www.healthline.com/human-body-maps/nasopharynx#1 — 11/1/22] For PDF, see Doc. Folder OAI53. "It contains adenoid tissue, which fights infection ..."

[82] IBID. Healthline Editorial Team ...

[83] IBID. Sanchez, Edith ... "Most of the mucus ... mixes with saliva and you swallow it. ... Then, when you sneeze or blow your nose, you get rid of the mucus." When we catch a cold, the body produces histamine that causes the production of more mucus. This causes you to need to blow your nose, or sneeze more often, which "helps expel the infectious agent."

[84] IBID. Sanchez, Edith ...

[85] IBID. Dhand, Rajiv and Li, Jie ... See under "Cough Stimulation of sensory nerve fibers ..." etc.

[86] IBID. Schwab, Jan-Alexander ...

Some of these particles between 0.3 and 0.5 μm might be captured by cilia in the upper branches of the bronchia in the lungs, and moved to the primary bronchus, at the trachea where they agitate a cough or swallow response to either eject the foreign particles from the body or neutralize them by digestion.[87] [88] [89] However, some particles, called "respirable aerosols," defined as particles that are ≤5 μm (up to 5000 nanometers), can reach the bronchiole and alveoli.[90] Most of the particles less than 0.5 μm (500 nm) will pass into the lower respiratory regions of the bronchioles — the very small passages that branch off the bronchi and deliver air to "tiny sacs called alveoli."[91]

The virus particles that elude the primary and secondary natural filtration defenses pass into the lungs, and those small enough to escape capture by the cilia move through the bronchia until they reach the alveoli.[92] Here, the invading virus particles encounter another immunity defense, where specialized cells

---

[87] Stannard, Wendy & O'Callaghan, Chris, *Ciliary function and the role of cilia in clearance,* NIH, National Library of Medicine, National Center for Biotechnology Information, PubMed.gov, 2006 [ONLINE: https://pubmed.ncbi.nlm.nih.gov/16551222/ — 11/2/22] For PDF, see Doc. Folder OAI54. The process is called "Mucociliary clearance," in which the mucus traps "inhaled particles and pathogens" and the cilia move the mucus with the trapped particles out of your lungs.

[88] Medical professional unnamed, *Bronchi,* published by Cleveland Clinic, last reviewed June 21, 2021 [ONLINE: https://my.clevelandclinic.org/health/body/21607-bronchi — 11/2/22] For PDF, see Doc. Folder OAI55. "The cilia help move mucus (phlegm) and particles out of your lungs. When you cough or swallow, the particles trapped in the mucus move out of your body or into your digestive tract, where your body can dispose of them."

[89] Dhand, Rajiv and Li, Jie, *Coughs and Sneezes: Their Role in Transmission of Respiratory Viral Infections, Including SARS-CoV-2,* American Journal of Respiratory and Critical Care Medicine, American Thoracic Society, June 16, 2020 [ONLINE: https://www.ncbi.nlm.nih.gov/pmc/articles/PMC7462404/#_ffn_sectitle — 10/29/22] For PDF, see Doc. Folder OAI51. "Particles >5 μm in aerodynamic diameter are most likely to deposit by impaction in the oropharynx and be swallowed."

[90] Milton, Donald K, MD, *A Rosetta Stone for Understanding Infectious Drops and Aerosols,* Journal of the Pediatric Infectious Diseases Society, Oxford University Press, September 2020 [ONLINE: https://www.ncbi.nlm.nih.gov/pmc/articles/ PMC7495905/#_ffn_sectitle — 11/2/22] For PDF, see Doc. Folder OR - FN01.38.00.03.28. (Milton received funding from NIAID and DARPA.)

[91] Eldridge, Lynne, MD, *The Anatomy of the Bronchioles,* verywellhealth/Anatomy, reviewed by Samad, Reza, MD, updated July 13, 2022 [ONLINE: https://www.verywellhealth.com/bronchioles-anatomy-function-and-diseases-2248931 — 11/2/22] For PDF, see Doc. Folder OAI56.

[92] IBID. Eldridge, Lynne, MD ...

attack them.[93] However, if the virions overwhelm this last defense, or the host's immunity is compromised and cannot mount an adequate defense, the infectious particle will enter the blood through the alveoli. [94] But the body does not give up. Other immunity responses occur within the blood to attack the foreign invaders. So, as you can see, God has created us to fight off any invasion of infectious particles, and we get sick only when that system breaks down. Masks, as I shall show below, actually facilitate the infectious particles in their invasion.

Masks aid and abet virus particle invasion.

Here is the problem with the mask: it captures and holds next to your face what your body is trying to eject. Whatever droplets it captures with any efficiency at all, would have been subject to capture by our natural filtration system, described above. However, your mask blocks the ≥5 μm droplet. Why is this a problem?

Depending on the force, or velocity of the droplet, when it hit your mask it was immediately broken down into smaller droplets. What comes next will shock most maskers.

If you are wearing a mask that includes what is called a hydrophobic (water resistant) filter, the droplet will break into smaller droplets upon impact. Depending on the momentum of the droplets upon impact they will 1. Remain trapped in the fibers until they desiccate (fully evaporate), or 2. Break into smaller droplets that will desiccate even more quickly, or 3. Push through the fibers of the mask. [95] The natural course of respiration, blowing and

---

[93] Naeem A, Rai SN, & Pierre L., *Histology, Alveolar Macrophages,* StatPearls Publishing, January 2022 [ONLINE: https://www.ncbi.nlm.nih.gov/books/NBK513313/#_NBK513313_pubdet_ — 11/2/22] For PDF, see Doc. Folder OAI58. "Alveolar macrophages (AM) also known as dust cells are a type of white blood cells. ... Alveolar macrophages are the first line of defense against invading respiratory pathogens."

[94] IBID. Dhand, Rajiv and Li, Jie ... see Figure 3. (You'll need to open the link found at Figure 3.)

[95] Aydin, Onur, et al., Performance of fabrics for homemade masks against the spread of COVID-19 through droplets: A quantitative mechanistic study, ScienceDirect, October 2020 [ONLINE: https://www.sciencedirect.com/science/article/pii/S2352431620301802 — 11/2/22] For PDF,

drawing air over the minute droplets, facilitates desiccation. Give it a hot day, or low humidity, the process is even faster, and soon the virion droplets are reduced to sizes that are either launched into aerosols in the atmosphere or drawn deep into your lungs. In this case, the virions FLY PAST YOUR NATURAL DEFENSES like a bee through a chain link fence.

If you are wearing what is called a hydrophilic (water absorbing) filter, it's even worse. Now the droplets absorb into the material, spreading out thinly over the surface, and so drying even more quickly, with the same result: the droplets shrink until they are launched from the mask into aerosols that move about with air currents indefinitely, or they are drawn past all your natural filtering barriers, deep into your bronchiole, through the opening into your alveoli; and if they survive the immune response of alveoli macrophage,[96] they enter into your blood cells where they begin replicating and causing infection.

Natural filtration is far superior to masks for protection against the public spread of viral infection. This does not mean masks should not be used for short duration in specific circumstances, for example, to protect a patient from a physician's ejecta getting into their open wounds. For general public use for hours at a time, and as protection from something so small as a virus, they are not only ineffective, they facilitate transmission, and cause multiple health concerns. [97]

---

see Doc. Folder OR - FN01.13.00.00.00. See 1. Results and discussion for a graphic illustration of what happens when a droplet impacts a mask.

[96] IBID. Naeem A, …

[97] Huber, Colleen NMD. Posted: *Masks Are Neither Effective Nor Safe: A Summary of the Science,* Citizens For Free Speech, July 15, 2020 [ONLINE: https://www.citizensforfreespeech.org/masks_are_neither_effective_nor_safe_a_summary_of_the_s cience — 11/17/22] For PDF, see Doc. Folder SEO13.00.00.00. (NOTE: In the End Notes, I discovered 4 duplicated articles, 1 retracted, 1 foreign language article, and one accessible with subscription only.) For 150 articles showing masks do not work to protect against the spread of a virus infection, see Doc. Folder SEO35.

Epilogue to the question of mask efficacy against a virus

So that's the science! To summarize: the only studies that seem to show support for masks are based on observational science. None of the studies used to support mask use for protection against public spread of a virus delivers! Not one! They typically fail to consider critical factors, like leakage, desiccation (evaporation), or they focus on particle sizes that are much larger than a virus particle, making the study irrelevant. Additionally, scientists don't put much confidence in these sorts of studies. Western scientists have depended upon Randomized Controlled Trials (RCTs) as the gold standard of scientific research. Every properly conducted RCT shows that masks are not an effective way to stop the spread of something so small as a virus. As for community protection, or *source control,* the mask only blocks larger virions that desiccate quickly and are either launched into the atmosphere as aerosols or drawn past all natural defenses deeply into the lower regions of the lungs where they can enter into the blood stream. It's Just like Fauci said in an email: "The typical mask you buy in the drug store is not really effective in keeping out virus, which is small enough to pass through the material."[98] But even worse, the masks Fauci, and the government medical establishment recommend actually facilitate viral infection.

---

[98] Howley, Patrick *Fauci Told Former Obama Admin Official In A Private Email: Don't Wear A Mask,* June 2, 2021 [ONLINE: https://nationalfile.com/fauci-told-former-obama-admin-official-in-a-private-email-dont-wear-a-mask/ — 11/17/22] For PDF, see Doc. Folder OAI93. For full quote, see article or find it quoted in full at Footnote 3.

Chapter Six:
Reasons we cannot trust the current government medical establishment

What is the government medical establishment?

I'll explain why I believe we cannot trust the medical establishment. But first, I need to define what I mean by the term. When I refer to the *government medical establishment*, I am talking about those employed in our government health departments. Of course, I can't know if every government-employed medical professional is untrustworthy. But the leadership knows the information I presented in previous chapters, so they are certainly culpable. Those down the chain of command are either too fearful to speak out or they accept without question the official position dictated to them by government "experts."

Fauci is presently (as of October 2022) at the head of the medical establishment. He is the highest-paid bureaucrat in the American government (400k+ p/y). His power and influence in the medical field of virology is pervasive. Some have facetiously claimed his power and influence exceed that of the President.[99]

The medical establishment also includes all private medical contractors connected to the government through grants or subsidies or whose employment/income is received substantially from the government. Many of these scientists are compromised by their dependency upon government funding for their research.

A second tier of what I call the *medical establishment* includes all medical persons who habitually depend on the government for guidance in their medical practice. Frankly, much of this arises

---

[99] Nelson, Steven, *Biden jokes Fauci is actual president as he shared COVID 'winter plan,'* December 2, 2021 [ONLINE: https://nypost.com/2021/12/02/biden-jokes-fauci-is-real-president-as-he-shares-covid-plan/ — 11/2/22] For PDF, see Doc. Folder OAI70. Even Biden recently joked that Fauci is the real POTUS.

from laziness on the part of some doctors and/or fatigue arising from the intensity of their professions.

There is a sort of invisible hierarchy in the medical profession, with Fauci at the top and the FDA and CDC serving as supports, combining the government's power of coercion with "scientific authority."

The CDC is a US government-funded agency that receives massive additional funding from Bill Gates and pharmaceutical companies, raising concerns about a conflict of interest.

Virtually all of the push for masking comes from this medical establishment, presently under the direction of Fauci.

Why we cannot trust the medical establishment today?

In today's politically charged environment, there is good reason to question whether the medical establishment is acting in the interests of the American people, or even in the interests of the science of medicine, but instead promoting some other agenda. Here is some of the evidence.

Remember that the consensus of western medicine recommended against use of masks as public policy for controlling the spread of a virus before the SARS-CoV-2 outbreak.

President Trump announced the appointment of Anthony Fauci to his "coronavirus task force" on January 29, 2020. [100] The President declared the Wuhan outbreak a public health emergency on January 31.[101] Then on February 5, 2020, Fauci sent an email to

---

[100] Behrmann, Savannah and Santucci, Jeanine, *Here's a timeline of President Donald Trump's and Dr. Anthony Fauci's relationship*, USA TODAY, October 28, 2020 [ONLINE: https://www.usatoday.com/story/news/politics/2020/10/28/president-donald-trump-anthony-fauci-timeline-relationship-coronavirus-pandemic/3718797001/ — 12/3/22] For PDF, see Doc. Folder OAI110.

[101] NCSL NATIONAL CONFERENCE OF STATE LEGISLATURES, Staff, *President Trump Declares State of Emergency for COVID-19*, NCSL, March 25, 2020 [ONLINE: https://www.ncsl.org/ncsl-in-dc/publications-and-resources/president-trump-declares-state-of-emergency-for-covid-19.aspx — 12/3/22] For PDF, see Doc. Folder OAI108.

Obama's former Health and Human Services Secretary, Sylvia Burwell, explaining, "The typical mask you buy in the drug store is not really effective in keeping out virus, which is small enough to pass through the material."[102] The US Surgeon General agreed, saying masks "are not effective in preventing [the] general public from catching #Coronavirus."[103] So did the CDC[104] and the World Health Organization (W.H.O.)[105] at first. So it's no surprise that every box of masks you buy has a disclaimer printed on it. Here is one example: "Masks are not designed or intended to prevent, mitigate, treat, diagnose or cure any disease or health condition, including COVID-19/Coronavirus."[106]

---

[102] Howley, Patrick, *Fauci Told Former Obama Admin Official In A Private Email: DON'T Wear A Mask,* National File, June 2, 2021 [ONLINE: https://nationalfile.com/fauci-told-former-obama-admin-official-in-a-private-email-dont-wear-a-mask/ — 11/2/22] For PDF, see Doc. Folder OAI59. Here is the full text of Dr. Fauci's email referenced in this article: "Sylvia: Masks are really for infected people to prevent them from spreading infection to people who are not infected [*source control*] rather than protecting uninfected people from acquiring infection. The typical mask you buy in the drug store is not really effective in keeping out virus, which is small enough to pass through the material. It might, however, provide some slight benefit in keep [sic] out gross droplets if someone coughs or sneezes on you. I do not recommend that you wear a mask, particularly since you are going to a very low risk location. Your instincts are correct, [sic - ;] money is best spent on medical countermeasures such as diagnostics and vaccines. Safe travels." (I address the question of *source control* thoroughly in Chapter Four.)

[103] Netburn, Deborah, *A timeline of the CDC's advice on face masks,* Los Angeles Times: Science & Medicine, July 27, 2021 [ONLINE: https://www.latimes.com/science/story/2021-07-27/timeline-cdc-mask-guidance-during-covid-19-pandemic — 12/3/22] For PDF, see Doc. Folder OAI111.

[104] IBID. Netburn, Deborah, A timeline of the CDC's advice on face masks …

[105] Howard, Jacqueline, *W.H.O. stands by recommendation to not wear masks if you are not sick or not caring for someone who is sick,* CNN, March 31, 2020 [ONLINE: https://www.cnn.com/2020/03/30/world/coronavirus-who-masks-recommendation-trnd/index.html — 12/3/22] For PDF, see Doc. Folder OAI113. By June of 2020, W.H.O. "fine-tunes advice on COVID masks for public …" See Nebehay, Stephanie, *W.H.O. fine-tunes advice on COVID masks for public, health workers,* Reuters, December 2, 2020 [ONLINE: https://www.reuters.com/article/uk-health-coronavirus-who-masks-idUKKBN28C170 — 12/3/22] For PDF, see Doc. Folder OAI114. By June of 2021, W.H.O. was recommending every one wear masks, even those who had been vaccinated: Chung, Gabrielle, *World Health Organization Urges Vaccinated People to Continue Wearing Masks Due to Delta Variant of COVID,* People: Lifestyle-Health, June 29, 2021 [ONLINE: https://people.com/health/who-urges-vaccinated-people-to-wear-masks-due-to-delta-variant/ — 12/3/22] For PDF, see Doc. Folder OAI115.

[106] TEEPUBLIC, *Masks—Legal Disclaimer for Customers,* nd [ONLINE: https://teepublic.zendesk.com/hc/en-us/articles/360047284753-Masks-Legal-Disclaimer-for-Customers — 11/2/22] For PDF, see Doc. Folder OAI68. Note: the N95 is the only mask rated to help block a particle as small as a virion (a complete infective form of a virus particle), but CDC expressly recommends against its use by the general public: see CANOPUS, *Disclaimer for face mask*

Yet, as if on cue, the CDC, the W.H.O., the US Surgeon General, and Fauci flipped on their position regarding masks, and have repeatedly declared masks help mitigate the spread of COVID-19.[107] According to Webster's Dictionary of the English Language, to *mitigate* means to "make less severe, intense, harsh, rigorous, painful," etc. Why would Fauci, the US Surgeon General, the CDC and the W.H.O. say masks don't work in February of 2020, and a few months later start insisting everyone wear them? [108]

Fauci scoffed at the suggestion that Americans would be wearing masks.[109] After he changed his mind about the value of masks to protect from a virus, the establishment media allowed

---

(N95), [ONLINE: https://www.canopusgroup.us/pages/disclaimer-for-face-mask-n95 — 11/2/22] For PDF, see Doc. Folder OAI69. The reason is 1. These need to be fitted professionally to provide the protection they offer, and 2. Medical professionals need these masks, and there is concern about general use creating a shortage.

[107] CDC publication, *Mitigation measures for COVID-19 in households and markets in non-US low-resource settings*, July 7, 2021. [ONLINE: https://www.cdc.gov/coronavirus/2019-ncov/global-covid-19/global-urban-areas.html — 11/17/22]. For PDF, see Doc. Folder OAI96. "Key points: To protect themselves and those around them from the spread of COVID-19 in densely populated neighborhoods and market settings, individuals can use personal controls such as **masking**, physical distancing, and ensuring proper ventilation." (Bold added for emphasis.) The mask manufacturers flatly contradict CDC, Fauci, et al.

[108] Perrett, Connor, *The US Surgeon General once warned against wearing face masks for the coronavirus but the CDC now recommends it,* INSIDER, March 2, 2020 [ONLINE: https://www.businessinsider.com/americans-dont-need-masks-pence-says-as-demand-increases-2020-2 — 11/2/22] For PDF, see Doc. Folder OAI61. A little over one month later, both Pence and the Surgeon General suddenly about faced, claiming "new information." The *newness* of the information is dubious. They were talking about asymptomatic transmission earlier (See Joseph, Andrew *Study Reports First Case of Coronavirus Spread by Asymptomatic Person,* Scientific American, January 2020 [ONLINE: https://www.scientificamerican.com/article/study-reports-first-case-of-coronavirus-spread-by-asymptomatic-person/ — 11/2/22] For PDF, see Doc. Folder OAI64. Later, *Scientific American* added an editor's note saying the story was based on "faulty information." However, the faulty information was not related to the report of asymptomatic spread. Reports about GHOST CARRIERS were circulating during the time Fauci, Pence, and the Surgeon General were warning the general public about dangers arising from wearing masks for protection against a virus. Fauci's explanation that he wanted to protect the mask supply for health workers is an admission he lied, that he manipulated the public. See Miltimore, Jon, *Fauci's Mask Flip-Flop, Explained (by Economics),* FEE Stories, June 3, 2021 [ONLINE: https://fee.org/articles/fauci-s-mask-flip-flop-explained-by-economics/ — 11/2/22] For PDF, see Doc. Folder OAI62.

[109] Cowhick, Jack, *Flashback: 1 Year Ago Fauci Said 'People Should Not Be Walking Around with Masks'* The Western Journal, March 8, 2021 [ONLINE: https://www.westernjournal.com/flashback-1-year-ago-fauci-said-people-not-walking-around-masks/ — 11/2/22] For PDF, see Doc. Folder OAI60.

him to explain. In his explanation, he admitted they are "largely symbolic."[110] Maybe that's why we have so many images of Fauci, and other leaders unmasked in public and around others. Rules for thee, but not for me?

Those telling us to wear the masks get irritated when we ask why they don't. San Francisco's Mayor, London Breed, attended a nightclub unmasked. When challenged, she said, "We don't need fun police to come in and micromanage and tell us what we should or shouldn't be doing."[111] I think many of us agree with the Mayor. But her actions say she does not believe masks protect against the spread of a virus. Indeed, from what we see, none of these people insisting we wear masks are afraid to go about in public without them. They don't believe their own hype! And more to our immediate point, we have no reason to trust them!

According to Fauci, to attack (question) him is to question *science* itself.[112] After Fauci's public statement to Rand Paul was met with increasing criticism, Fauci attempted to explain it away by asserting his positions changed with the science, and doubled down on his claim that to question him is tantamount to

---

[110]Creed, Wayne (Current online version removes Author) *Fauci says Masks largely symbolic, 2nd wave of corona may not happen*, Cape Charles Mirror, May 31, 2020 [ONLINE: http://www.capecharlesmirror.com/news/fauci-says-masks-largely-symbolic-2nd-wave-of-corona-may-not-happen/ — 11/17/22] For PDF, see Doc. Folder OAI16.

[111]CBS Bay Area, editorial: *San Francisco Mayor Defends Criticism After Video Catches Her Dancing Maskless at Night Club,* September 20, 2021 [ONLINE: https://sanfrancisco.cbslocal.com/2021/09/20/san-francisco-mayor-london-breed-defends-criticism-after-video-dancing-maskless-night-club/ — 11/2/22] For PDF, see Doc. Folder OAI63. (The hypocrisy of the "elites" is a clear proof they know the masks are useless).

[112] Aitken, Peter & Brown, Jon, *Rand Paul blasts Fauci: 'Astounding and alarming' to declare 'I represent science'* FoxNews, November 28, 2021 [ONLINE: https://www.foxnews.com/politics/rand-paul-blasts-fauci-astounding-alarming-represent-science — 11/3/22] For PDF, see Doc. Folder OAI72. In a Senate HELP Committee hearing, Rand Paul challenged Fauci over his flip-flopping messaging about mandates, "including mask-wearing"; Fauci retaliated by scolding Paul saying that because he, Dr. Fauci, represents science, to attack him "is really to attack science."

questioning science. [113] Really? The "science" changed? When? Where is the RCT that showed western science has been wrong about mask efficacy against a virus?

Here is another good reason we do not trust medical scientists today.[114] Fauci's colleague, Dr Collins, is Director of the National Institutes for Health (NIH); NIH has published articles asserting RCTs are the gold standard for medical research.[115] [116] Fauci has more than once declared them to be the "gold standard" of scientific research.[117] For example, he insisted upon RCTs when criticizing calls for the use of Hydroxychloroquine (HCQ) as early treatment for COVID-19. He repeatedly explained his reason was there were no RCTs supporting its use for COVID. When asked why Fauci "felt so strongly about the trials," he answered, "Well, because it is the gold standard," and explained, "you have to compare your intervention with something. Because the medical literature and experience is full of situations of anecdotal

---

[113] Brown, Lee, *Fauci doubles down on claim that attacks on him are 'actually criticizing science'*, New York Post, June 21, 2021 [ONLINE: https://nypost.com/2021/06/21/fauci-attacks-on-him-are-actually-criticizing-science/ — 11/3/22] For PDF, see Doc. Folder OAI73.

[114] It's beyond the scope of this book, but if you have studied the controversy in the science community over global warming, you find all the same elements of politicization that you find in medical science today.

[115] Hariton, Eduardo, MD, MBA & Locascio, Joseph J. PhD, *Randomized controlled trials—the gold standard for effectiveness research*, BJOG: an international journal of obstetrics and gynaecology [European spelling], Published NIH, June 19. 2018 [ONLINE: https://www.ncbi.nlm.nih.gov/pmc/articles/PMC6235704/#_ffn_sectitle — 11/3/22] For PDF, see Doc. Folder OAI78.

[116] Kabisch, Maria, et al., *Randommised Controlled Trials*, Deutsches Arzteblatt International, translated from German by David Roseveare, September 30, 2011 [ONLINE: https://www.ncbi.nlm.nih.gov/pmc/articles/PMC3196997/#_ffn_sectitle — 11/3/22] For PDF, see Doc. Folder OAI79. "Randomized controlled clinical trials (RCTs) are the gold standard for ascertaining the efficacy and safety of a new treatment ..." or intervention, "Since RCTs are by definition interventional, often investigating drugs or medical devices ..." such as masks.

[117] Lurie, Peter, MD, MPH, *My interview with Dr. Anthony Fauci*, Center For Science In the Public Interest, updated: December 29, 2020 [ONLINE: https://www.cspinet.org/news/beyond-the-curve/interview-dr-anthony-fauci — 11/3/22] For PDF, see Doc Folder OAI74. Dr. Lurie asked how was the vaccines' effectiveness determined? Fauci replied: "By state-of-the-art, gold standard, randomized placebo-controlled trials."

retrospective cohort studies that have proven to be wrong."[118] Okay, so where are the RCTs that support his claim that the science has changed regarding masks? *Crickets!* Fauci has never directed us to any RCT that supports surgical and/or cloth masks as effective to control the public spread of a virus for personal or for community protection.

There are no randomized controlled trials that support Fauci's mask recommendations. In fact, there are no comprehensive scientific experiments that take into consideration all the factors involved in mask efficacy (penetration, leakage, droplet desiccation, viral load for infection, etc.) that show any change in the established science regarding masks. As I show in my extensive research, after examining more than 500 scientific articles purporting to prove masks work, every one of them is a species of observational science, based on anecdotal, retrospective, and cohort studies, or a combination thereof — studies that Fauci dismissed as inadequate to support any scientific conclusion. The fact is, if you *follow the science,* you will see that the surgical or cloth masks recommended by establishment medical professionals will not provide adequate protection from transmission for the wearer or for the community.

Fauci telling Senator Paul that to question him is to question science is laughable, and only slightly more bizarre than it is ridiculous. Science is the accumulation of knowledge based on conclusions derived from observations tested through carefully controlled experiments. These experiments must be made public and verifiable by any who may replicate the experiment. The RCT is the gold standard. But we are noticing some establishment scientists beginning to challenge the value of randomized

---

[118] Rodack, Jeffrey, *Fauci Disputes Yale Doctor on Hydroxychloroquine Trials,* Newsmax, August 6, 2020 [ONLINE: https://www. newsmax.com/newsfront/fauci-risch-hydroxychloroquine-trials/2020/08/06/id/980862/ — 11/3/22] For PDF, see Doc. Folder OAI76.

controlled trials.[119] Here is a PubMed.gov article titled *Challenging the hegemony of randomized controlled trials: A commentary on Deaton and Cartwright.*[120]

Fauci seems to be the point man leading medical science away from empirically tested evidence-based scientific conclusions (consistent with the traditions of western science) to *scientism,* which is based on the pronouncements of scientists that are premised on the sort of "evidence" used to support mere superstitions. *Scientism* is the new *priestcraft,* and Fauci seems to be the current high priest! Fauci *speaks for science,* so what he says *is science?* We must reject this new cult! *Science* is not the mere statement of a scientist.

For example, the following from an article in the New England Journal of Medicine is not a *scientific* statement: "As SARS-CoV-2 continues its global spread, it's *possible* that one of the pillars of Covid-19 pandemic control — universal facial masking — *might* help reduce the severity of disease and ensure that a greater proportion of new infections are asymptomatic."[121] (Italics added

---

[119]Mulder, Roger, et al., *The limitations of using randomized controlled trials as a basis for developing treatment guidelines*, NIH National Library of Medicine, National Center for Biotechnology Information, PubMed.gov, July 14, 2017 [ONLINE: https://pubmed.ncbi.nlm.nih.gov/28710065/ — 11/3/22] For PDF, see Doc. Folder OAI80. The recent behaviour of Fauci, the CDC, and W.H.O. is causing some to ask whether RCTs continue to be the "gold standard." Beaman, Jeremy, Energy and Environment Reporter, *Are randomized controlled trials no longer the 'gold standard'?* Washington Examiner, February 1, 2021 [ONLINE: https://www.washingtonexaminer.com/opinion/are-randomized-controlled-trials-no-longer-the-gold-standard — 11/3/22] For PDF, see Doc. Folder OAI75.

[120] Pearl, Judea, affiliated with the University of CA, *Challenging the hegemony of randomized controlled trials: A commentary on Deaton and Cartwright,* NIH National Library of Medicine, National Center for Biotechnology Information, PubMed.gov, April 17, 2018 [ONLINE: https://pubmed.ncbi.nlm.nih.gov/29704961/ — 11/3/22] For PDF, see Doc. Folder OAI81.

[121] Gahnhi, Monica MD, MPH, and Rutherford, George W. MD, *Facial Masking for Covid-19 — Potential for "Variolation" as We Await a Vaccine,* The New England Journal of Medicine, Perspective, October 29, 2020 [ONLINE: https://www.nejm.org/doi/pdf/10.1056/NEJMp2026913?listPDF=true — 4/15/21] For PDF, see Doc. Folder OAI97. (As you read this article note the use of such expressions as the following (Italics added for emphasis): "*If* this hypothesis is borne out," "masking *seemed* to be a possible way," "*suggested* ... a strong relationship between public masking and pandemic control," "facial masking *may* also reduce ... ," and "The *possibility* is consistent with a long-standing *theory* of viral pathogenesis," "*If* the viral inoculum (— volume of virions present, ed.) matters ... an additional *hypothesized* reason ... ," "masking *might*

for emphasis.) Such a statement is an opinion that perhaps reflects the views of some scientists. But such *declarations,* even when made by scientists, are not by themselves *science.* Scientists are human and susceptible to bias, blackmail, bullying and other motivations to make assertions that are not supported by *science.*

Here is another dramatic example of political bias in the medical establishment. On March 19, Trump suggested use of hydroxychloroquine (HCQ) as a possible treatment for COVID-19. He heard from medical professionals that it was being used effectively, and said, "We should give it a try."[122] The President was viciously attacked for his suggestion, ridiculed, and mocked. Soon after, a "scientific" study was published in *The Lancet* alleging HCQ was ineffective and dangerous for use against COVID-19. *The Lancet* is a weekly peer-reviewed medical journal, considered to be the world's most impactful academic journal of its kind. So it scandalized that 200-year-old respected journal when the article turned out to be a lie![123]

---

reduce the (—volume of virions, ed.) that an exposed person inhales," and "*might* contribute." The idea that "*if* this theory bears out," and something *could* and *might* reduce infection and transmission, it should therefore be tried is very short sighted. No consideration is given to the number of deaths by suicide arising from despair caused by the lockdowns, which are associated with the masking strategy, together with the sometimes severe reactions of some vulnerable persons to wearing masks for extended periods, such as that addressed in the respected Journal of Primary Care & Community Health article titled, *The Effects of the Face Mask on the Skin Underneath: A Prospective Survey During the COVID-19 Pandemic*, first published October 21, 2020 (authors and contributors are identified by initials only). And then there are the multiple challenges coming against the official narrative arising from more current data: "asymptomatic infection rates are reported to be higher than 80% in settings with universal facial masking." Assertions that "Countries that have adopted population-wide masking have fared better ..." are challenged by more up to date data that informs us States that have removed lockdowns and masking mandates are faring better than those that continue those extreme mitigation strategies.

[122] Solender, Andrew, Forbes Staff, *All The Times Trump Has Promoted Hydroxychloroquine,* Forbes, May 22, 2020 [ONLINE: https://www.forbes.com/sites/andrewsolender/2020/05/22/all-the-times-trump-promoted-hydroxychloroquine/?sh=6067c8524643 — 12/21/22] For PDF, see Doc. Folder OAI118. Mr. Solender makes a reference to the "new study [that] found [HCQ] is linked to an increased risk of death in patients." His statement is linked to the retracted Lancet study, undermining Mr. Solender, Forbes, Lancet, Fauci, and all the others who used this fake study to attack Trump politically.

[123] Justice, Tristan, *Lancet Formally Retracts Fake Hydroxychloroquine Study Used By Media To Attack Trump,* The Federalist, June 4, 2020 [ONLINE: https://thefederalist.com/2020/06/04/lancet-formally-retracts-fake-hydroxychloroquine-study-

The World Health Organization (W.H.O.) admitted they discouraged using hydroxychloroquine (HCQ) to treat COVID patients based on the fake study published in *The Lancet* May 22, 2020.[124] Yet the scandal has gotten so little exposure in the EM (Establishment Media, aka, Main Stream Media, aka the Legacy Media) that many Americans continue to be ignorant that the study was proven to be fake science. *The Lancet* website published the formal retraction statement of three of its four authors, and marked the study RETRACTED, June 13, 2020.[125] Richard Horton, editor in chief of *The Lancet* described the article as "a monumental fraud." [126] *Monumental,* indeed! Keep in mind that this study provided the authority of *science* used by the government medical establishment, and politicians to prohibit the use of HCQ as early COVID-19 treatment with the quiet acquiescence of Fauci.

Indeed, Dr. Fauci, who had resisted calls for the use of HCQ in the early treatment of COVID, on May 27, 2020, a few days after the Lancet study was published, alluded to this study in his recommendations against use of HCQ for COVID.[127] I can't find that

---

used-by-media-to-attack-trump-inbox/ — 11/3/22] For PDF, see Doc. Folder OAI29b. To read the original Lancet study, see Mehra, Mandeep, R. MD, Desai, Sapan S. MD, Ruschitzka, Frank, Prof. MD, Patel, Amit N. MD, *RETRACTED: Hydroxychloroquine or chloroquine with or without a macrolide for treatment of COVID-19: a multinational registry analysis,* May 22, 2020 [ONLINE: https://www.thelancet.com/journals/lancet/article/PIIS0140-6736%2820%2931180-6/fulltext — 11/3/22] For PDF, see Doc. Folder OAI77.

[124] IBID Justice, Tristan …

[125] Mehra, Mandeep R., Ruschitzka, Frank, & Patel, Amit N. *Retraction—Hydroxychloroquine or chloroquine with or without macrolide for treatment of COVID-19: a multinational registry analysis,* originally published in THE LANCET, May 22, 2020, retracted June 13, 2020 [ONLINE: https://www.thelancet.com/journals/lancet/article/PIIS0140-6736(20)31324-6/fulltext — 11/12/22] For PDF, see Doc. Folder OAI84. The authors of this retraction are three of the original four authors of the original article. Their statement, in part: "After publication of our Lancet Article [named above], several concerns were raised with respect to the veracity of the data and analyses conducted by Surgisphere Corporation and its founder and our co-author, Sapan Desai, in our publication."

[126] Knight, Sam, *The Lancet Editor's Wild Ride Through the Coronavirus Pandemic,* The New Yorker, June 27, 2020 [ONLINE: https://www.newyorker.com/news/letter-from-the-uk/the-lancet-editors-wild-ride-through-the-coronavirus-pandemic — 3/15/23] For PDF, see OAI123.

[127] POLITICO, *Fauci: Hydroxychloroquine not effective against coronavirus,* POLITICO (includes video clip) May 27, 2020 [ONLINE: https://www.politico.com/news/2020/05/27/fauci-hydroxychloroquine-not-effective-against-coronavirus-283980 — 11/12/22] For PDF, see Doc.

Fauci has ever acknowledged the study was not authentic and that it was debunked as fake. Nor can I find that he has retracted his negative statements against the use of HCQ for early treatment. How can we trust such dishonest people?

The one mask that might block something as small as a virus particle is the N95.[128] But that's the mask Fauci and the CDC repeatedly say we should not use. The establishment medical professionals don't recommend the N95 because while they are rated to block well over 90% of particles as small as 100 nanometers,[129] they don't work unless carefully fitted. Even then, the seal is easily compromised, which requires refitting. Additionally, no one recommends wearing these masks for more

---

Folder OAI85. Previously, Fauci had made repeated statements declaring no RCTs showed HCQ efficacy against COVID, but never suggested its use could cause serious adverse reactions. However, about five days after the *Lancet* study was published, and had gained widespread circulation, and was being cited as evidence HCQ could cause serious adverse reactions in COVID patients, such as cardio vascular problems and Arrhythmia, Anthony Fauci made a statement you can listen to at the video linked above. In that statement, Fauci said, "The scientific data is really quite evident *now* about the lack of efficacy for it, and even the possibility that there could be, not could be, but there's, you know, a likelihood, that under certain circumstances, it might be rare, but you'd see it, adverse events, particularly with regard to cardio vascular and the arrhythmias that might be associated with it; I mean there was suspicion of that for a while, but as data comes in, it becomes more clear..." Fauci clearly claimed that HCQ could be dangerous when used to treat COVID-19, and the context of his statement makes it clear he was referring to the *Lancet* study.

[128] OSHA Review, Blog: *OSHA Requirements for Occupational Use of N95 Respirators in Healthcare,* OSHA Review, April 28, 2020 [ONLINE: https://oshareview.com/2020/04/osha-requirements-for-occupational-use-of-n95-respirators-in-healthcare/ — 11/2/22] For PDF, see Doc. Folder TECH75. "When worn properly (with the mask making a tight seal with the user's face), surgical N95 masks can filter at least 95% of very small (0.3 micron) test particles." The seal is critical to achieving this result. The SARS-CoV-2 virus particles are reported to range from ~70-170 nm (including the spike proteins), and the N95 is tested against particles that are 300 nm.

[129] Qian, Y, et al., *Performance of N95 respirators: filtration efficiency for airborne microbial and inert particles,* NIH, National Library of Medicine, PubMed.gov, February 1998 [ONLINE: https://pubmed.ncbi.nlm.nih. gov/9487666/ — 11/2/22] For PDF, see Doc. Folder OAI65. The most penetrating particle size for the N95 is 0.1 to 0.3 μm (100-300 nm), but according to Qian, Y et al., all the N95s tested were "at least 95% efficient at that size range for NaCI particles." This puts the N95 as efficient to capture particles at least within the range of SARS-CoV-2 particles. For discussion re SARS-CoV-2 particle size, see IBID. Na Zhu, Ph.D., et al., *A Novel Coronavirus from Patients with Pneumonia in China*, New England Journal of Medicine, January 24, 2020 [ONLINE: https://www.nejm.org/doi/10.1056/NEJMoa2001017 — 9/25/22] For PDF, see Doc. Folder OR - FN01.37.01.02.00.

than a few hours at a time.[130] Many cannot tolerate them for more than thirty minutes to an hour, especially during exertion.[131]

That leaves us with your typical *surgeon's* mask or cloth masks. We've discussed these above: the science does not support using these masks for protection against viral transmission or contagion.

The FDA, and the W.H.O. are aware of the above information. We already read Fauci's email betraying his knowledge of this before the pandemic. What about the CDC?

A May 2020 study published by the CDC concluded: "In our systematic review, we identified 10 RCTs [Randomized Controlled Trials] that reported estimates of the effectiveness of face masks in reducing laboratory-confirmed influenza virus infections in the community from literature published during 1946-July 27, 2018. In pooled analysis, we found NO SIGNIFICANT REDUCTION IN INFLUENZA TRANSMISSION WITH THE USE OF FACE MASKS."[132]

---

[130] Bielcor (manufacturer), *How Long Can You Wear An N95 Mask?* Bielcor, November 25, 2021 [ONLINE: https://www.bielcor.com/ how-long-can-you-wear-an-n95-mask/ — 11/2/22] For PDF, see Doc. Folder OAI66. Note: it's often true that you will get more honest assessments of product use from the manufacturer than from CDC. This is because CDC bears ZERO liability for their recommendations and is a highly politicized government subsidized institution. For example, in Bielcor's statement, notice that under the subheading *How Long Can You Wear An N95 Mask?* you read the following: "The official statement from the CDC is that healthcare workers can wear an N95 mask for up to eight consecutive hours. That does not mean it is smart or recommended to wear them for that long without changing them. Though it is possible in an emergency and when seriously limited amounts of masks are available." Then read the summary: "How long can you wear an N95 mask? Masks should only be worn for a few hours at a time." People who are using these masks for 4-8 hours a day and the same mask for a week or weeks at a time are fooling themselves if they think they are providing adequate protection for themselves or their neighbours. Example, touch the mask one time and you are encouraged to change it. The seal on these is easily compromised and when that happens, the N95 performs no better than a typical surgical or cloth mask.

[131] California Department of Public Health, *Emergency Preparedness Office (EPO): N95 Respiratory Masks FAQs,* FDA, updated October 29, 2019 [ONLINE: https://www.cdph.ca.gov/Programs/EPO/Pages/Wildfire%20Pages/N95-Respirators-FAQs.aspx — 11/2/22] For PDF, see Doc. Folder OAI67. "Q. Will wearing an N95 respirator make it hard to breathe normally? A: N95 respirators may make breathing more difficult and lead to increased breathing and heart rates."

[132] Xiao, Jingyi; Shiu, Eunice Y.C., et al. *Nonpharmaceutical Measures for Pandemic Influenza in Nonhealthcare Personal Protective and Environmental Measures,* CDC, Emerging Infectious Diseases, Volume 26, Number 5—May 2020 [ONLINE: https://wwwnc.cdc.gov/eid/article/26/5/19-0994_article — 3/25/23] For PDF, see Doc. Folder OAI21.01.811.17.2. Note: This article explains

In other words, five months into the pandemic, the CDC looked for any RCT research that supported using masks and couldn't find any. The reason is that flu (or influenza) virus particles are between 80 and 120 nanometers. The openings in a surgical mask are 300 nanometers. The typical cloth masks have openings that range from 80 to 500 μm (80,000 to 500,000 nm).[133] By the way, remember the virus causing COVID-19 is ~70-170 nm.[134] Do the math!

So what accounts for the dramatic change in the *opinions* of *some* medical professionals? Let's just say, "the love of money is the root of all evil"[135] and the thief comes only to "steal, kill, and destroy." [136] Whatever agenda the medical establishment is pushing, it's not about science, and it's not about health. And at this point, we cannot trust them.

---

that "Disposable medical masks (also known as surgical masks) are loose-fitting devices that were designed to be worn by medical personnel to protect [against] accidental contamination of patient wounds, and to protect the wearer against splashes or sprays of bodily fluids."

[133] Bhakta, Bhana, et al., *Optical microscopic study of surface morphology and filtering efficiency of face masks,* PeerJ, The Open Access journal for Life & Environment research, June 26, 2019 [ONLINE: https://www.ncbi.nlm.nih.gov/pmc/articles/ PMC6599448/#_ffn_sectitle — 11/2/22] For PDF, see Doc. Folder OAI71. These researchers examined typical low cost cloth masks and found the average pore size to be "from 80 to 500 μm." See under *Results*.

[134] IBID: Na Zhu, Ph.D., et al., *A Novel Coronavirus ...*

[135] 1Timothy 6:10 (KJV)

[136] John 10:10 (KJV)

Chapter Seven:
The Documentation

What do we find in the studies that show masks do not work?

Many experiments have been done to determine whether or not masks effectively protect wearers from the transmission or contagion of diseases caused by a virus. The best method used to identify what causes a disease is called Randomized Controlled Trials (RCTs). I provide access to several of these studies in the footnote below, [137] and more than 140 articles detailing the science that says masks do not provide adequate protection from virus in my supplement Doc. Folder SE-Supporting Evidence. [138] I will provide a summary overview of what you will find as you examine that material:

First, the only masks that might provide some meaningful protection are the masks all medical establishment professionals are telling the public not to wear—the N95.[139]

Second, you will find that surgical masks do not provide an effective barrier to virus infection. I addressed this in great detail earlier. In summary: it's obvious that a particle that is ~70-170 nm

---

[137] Posted by Colleen Huber, NMD, via PrimaryDoctor, *Masks Are Neither Effective Nor Safe: A Summary of the Science,* Technocracy News & Trends, July 14, 2020 [ONLINE: https://www.technocracy.news/masks-are-neither-effective-nor-safe-a-summary-of-the-science/ — 11/2/22] For PDF, see Doc. Folder SEO13.00.00.00. (NOTE: During my examination of Huber's post, I discovered 4 duplicated articles, 1 retracted, 1 foreign language article, and one accessible with subscription only.) For over 140 articles, including a few audio recordings, showing masks do not work to protect against the spread of a virus infection, see Doc. Folder SE-Supporting Evidence - Research Supporting My Thesis.

[138] The Supplemental Material is available free with the purchase of this book. Go to www.booksatdbp.com and use the coupon code LMPB-1 at checkout.

[139] Parker, TJ, *CDC does not recommend general public wear N95's, here's why,* Eyewitness News, ABC, January 28, 2021 [ONLINE: https://abc7ny.com/n95-mask-cdc-recommendation-dr-rochelle-walensky-what-type-of-is-the-best/10092451/ — 11/17/22] For PDF, see Doc. Folder OAI98. "Dr. Walensky [CDC-Director], as well as Dr. Anthony Fauci, are still saying people should wear a mask, but say the general public doesn't need to wear the N95 ones because they're uncomfortable and hard to breathe in."

easily penetrates a mask with pores that are 300-50,000 nm. For this reason, more current studies concentrate on the droplets that carry the virus particles, which are larger than 300 nm to 5 μm (5000 nm). But as you research, you'll see that the virus easily escapes through the mask as the droplet evaporates, which, in almost every case, occurs within seconds.

Third, you will discover that, although cloth masks are virtually worthless for protection, according to some scientists, they are helpful for two things. 1. They provide emotional security to the wearer and the frightened public. (I think they would have done more to assuage fear by using their erstwhile-enjoyed reputation with the American people to tell them the truth about the threat of COVID and the inadequacy of masks.) And 2. They remind people that there is a pandemic and heightened awareness encourages carefulness in other ways: washing hands, social distancing, etc. In other words, our presumptuous masters decided to use masks for manipulating the public and promoting fear.

I don't know about you, but it insults me that these arrogant people use deceit and manipulation to control our behavior. Please understand that the reason they must resort to these devious methods is that the truth interferes with their agenda, which is control of public behavior, and they cannot provide factual, real science to support the recommendations and mandates they use to extend that control over the public.

Fourth, when you compare pre-COVID, COVID, and post-COVID studies, you will find that the science in all the RCTs is virtually the same. By *the science*, I mean the methods used and the documented test results achieved. However, a change occurs in the recommendations and conclusions of the scientists.

Before COVID-19, no western scientist concluded in favor of masks as public policy.[140] During the early stages of the COVID outbreak, scientists concluded similarly.

---

[140] Rancourt, Dennis G. *Masks Don't Work: A Review of Science Relevant to COVID-19 Social Policy,* River Cities Reader, June 11, 2020 [ONLINE: https://www.rcreader.com/commentary/masks-dont-work-covid-a-review-of-science-relevant-to-covide-19-social-policy — 11/16/22] For PDF, see Doc. Folder SE026. Most of the studies cited are pre-COVID: Jacobs, Joshua L. et al., 2009 *Use of surgical face masks to reduce the incidence of the common cold among health care workers in Japan: A randomized controlled trial,* American Journal of Infection Control (AJIC), Brief Report, Vol. 37, Issue 5, June 1, 2009 [ONLINE: paid access: https://www.ajicjournal.org/article/S0196-6553(08)00909-7/fulltext — 11/15/22] For PDF, see Doc. Folder SE027. Cowling, B. J. et al., *Face masks to prevent transmission of influenza virus: a systematic review,* Cambridge University Press, January 22, 2010 [ONLINE:https://www.cambridge.org/core/journals/epidemiology-and-infection/article/face-masks-to-prevent-transmission-of-influenza-virus-a-systematic-%20review/64D368496EBDE0AFCC6639CCC9D8BC05 — 11/15/22] For PDF, see Doc. Folder SE028. "None of the studies reviewed showed a benefit from wearing a mask, in either HCW (Health Care Worker) or community members in households (H)." bin-Reza, Faisal et al., *The use of masks and respirators to prevent transmission of influenza: a systematic review of the scientific evidence,* December 21, 2011 [ONLINE: https://onlinelibrary.wiley.com/doi/epdf/10.1111/j.1750-2659.2011.00307.x — 11/15/22] For PDF, see Doc. Folder SE029.00. "There were 17 eligible studies, ... None of the studies established a conclusive relationship between mask/respirator use and protection against influenza infection." Smith, Jeffery D. et al, *Effectiveness of N95 respirators versus surgical masks in protecting health care workers from acute respiratory infection: a systematic review and meta-analysis,* Canadian Medical Association Journal (CMAJ), May 17, 2016 [ONLINE: https://www.cmaj.ca/content/188/8/567 — 11/15/22] For PDF, see Doc. Folder SE029.01. This study is limited to an examination of relative protection between N95 and surgical face masks. Offeddu, Vittoria et al., *Effectiveness of Masks and Respirators Against Respiratory Infections in Healthcare Workers: A Systematic Review and Meta-Analysis,* August 7, 2017 [ONLINE: https://academic.oup.com/cid/article/65/11/1934/4068747?login=false — 11/15/22] For PDF, see Doc. Folder SE030. "Evidence of a protective effect of masks or respirators against verified respiratory infection (VRI) was not statistically significant." Radonovich, Lewis J. et al., *N95 Respirators vs Medical Masks for Preventing Influenza Among Health Care Personnel,* September 3, 2019 [ONLINE: https://jamanetwork.com/journals/jama/fullarticle/2749214 — 11/15/22] For PDF, see Doc. Folder SE031. "...N95 respirators vs. medical masks as worn by [2371] participants in this trial resulted in no significant difference in the incidence of laboratory-confirmed influenza." NOTE: Keep in mind the studies we have already examined that prove surgical masks do not protect against infection. Then we come to 2020: Long, Youlin et al. *Effectiveness of N95 respirators versus surgical masks against influenza: A systematic review and meta-analysis,* February 3, 2020 [ONLINE: https://onlinelibrary. wiley.com/doi/epdf/ 10.1111/jebm.12381 — 11/15/22] For PDF, see Doc. Folder SE032. "A total of six RCTs involving 9,171 participants were included. There were no statistically significant differences in preventing laboratory-confirmed influenza, laboratory-confirmed respiratory viral infections, laboratory-confirmed respiratory infection, and influenza-like illness using N95 respirators AND SURGICAL MASKS." (Emphasis added.) These studies show that even the much-vaulted N95 does not afford adequate protection against a viral infection. Conclusion: "No RCT study with verified outcome shows a benefit for HCW or community members in households to wearing a mask or respirator. There is NO SUCH STUDY, THERE ARE NO EXCEPTIONS." (Emphasis added.)

But a change occurred a few months into the declared pandemic. The science did not change, but scientists' conclusions started changing. First, I noticed statements like masks *could* help, *might* help, and they *possibly provide some mitigation value*, and so on began to appear. Then, as Fauci and others insisted on masks and politicians started calling for mask mandates, scientists began including in their summaries remarks such as *masks are required by...*, and *CDC says*, and so on.

Finally, you will notice that multiple post-COVID RCT studies examined the question of mask efficacy against virus, but these showed no appreciable change in results from similar pre-COVID RCTs. Nonetheless, after the pandemic got underway, the conclusions began to change. At first, they would stipulate the science showed no appreciable protection was afforded by use of masks, but added that the CDC or the W.H.O. recommends them. Then they started stating in their conclusions that masks *might* afford *some* protection. Finally, even though the science represented in the RCT actually provided no support for recommending masks, in the conclusions of some studies I began to notice firm recommendations for mask use as public policy. It was becoming increasingly clear that political pressure was affecting these scientists.

In addition, I noticed that the research showed increasing CCP influence. On the question of the efficacy of masks as public policy to control the spread of a virus, there is a discernible transition from traditional western medical science recommending against masks toward eastern medical science that favors them. Particularly troubling was the noticeable shift toward reliance upon the studies created by CCP (Chinese Communist Party) controlled medicine.[141] Science in a free society is practiced very differently than in controlled communities, like China under the

---

[141] Review my chronological arrangement of the hundreds of articles and studies I examined for this book: Doc. Folder OR Research CHRONOLOGICAL TABLE. You will notice this trend as you examine CCP: authors, origins, references, and funding.

CCP. Happily, some medical scientists began to resist the government-controlled narrative and expose the fake science used to support it.[142]

I should point out that researchers have given up trying to support mask use with RCTs—regarded as the *gold standard of scientific research to test medical interventions, like masks*. It has become popular to cite *observational studies* to show *scientific* support for their use. However, observational studies are considered inadequate to support firm conclusions regarding treatment protocols and serious scientists continue to distrust them.

What about the study that showed masks can block particles as small as 50 nanometers in size? (An example of "scientific sleight of hand")

I picked this study to illustrate why it is important to read these research articles carefully. In Footnote No. 1, you will find a link to what I call the *Falcon 49*, where Mr. Falcon cites 49 studies used to support wearing masks as public policy to control the spread of a virus. One of those studies appears to argue that masks can block particles as small as 50 nanometers. [143] That's a startling claim.

As I pointed out earlier, none of the studies in the *Falcon 49* is a valid RCT. This study is not an exception. However, superficially read, some might think this study proves masks work against particles as small as 0.05 μm (50 nm). It was published by the

---

[142] LifeSite *News* editorial: *Physicians: 'Masks don't control viruses, they control you,' 'pandemic is over,'* LifeSiteNews, October 29, 2020 [ONLINE: https://www.lifesitenews.com/news/group-of-doctors-masks-are-completely-irrelevant-to-blocking-covid-19 — 11/15/22] For PDF, see Doc. Folder SE034. See especially, Alexander, Paul E., *More than 150 Comparative Studies and Articles on Mask **Ineffectiveness and Harms**,* Brownstone Institute, [Emphasis added.] December 20, 2021 [ONLINE: https://brownstone.org/articles/more-than-150-comparative-studies-and-articles-on-mask-ineffectiveness-and-harms/ — 11/15/22] For PDF, see Doc. Folder SE035.

[143] Clapp, Phillip W. et al. Evaluation of Cloth Masks and Modified Procedure Masks as Personal Protective Equipment for the Public During the COVID-19 Pandemic, JAMA Internal Medicine, December 10, 2020 [ONLINE: https://jamanetwork.com/ journals/jamainternalmedicine/article-abstract/2774266 — 11/15/22] For PDF, see Doc. Folder OAI87. See also Doc. Folder OR - FN01.16.00.00.00.

reputable *Journal of the American Medical Association* (JAMA) and so the first question is why wouldn't Fauci, et al, be pushing this study front-and-center in this debate? It turns out, there is a very good reason they don't.

The study interested me because it tested for particles as small as 50 nanometers and insinuated surgical masks provide some appreciable protection if "simple modifications" are used. [144] However, a close reading reveals that they achieved their results using special electret filter media (electrostatically charged material), as opposed to material designed to protect against aerodynamic, or free floating particles, such as the common "nonelectret" surgical and cloth mask we are counseled to wear. According to this study, these "nonelectret filter media" masks are penetrated by particles as large as 200 to 300 nanometers. Remember, SARS-CoV-2 particles range from ~70-170 nm. Here we have a study purporting to prove masks are effective to protect against virus infection that actually proves the masks we are told to wear do not work. You have to read these studies carefully and pay attention.

The researchers stipulated other limitations that virtually disqualify this study from being useful in this debate. For example, they used only one test subject and the masks tested were very carefully fitted to that subject's face. The wide variation in facial structure makes this study virtually meaningless of any practical value with regard to the question whether masks should be mandated for prevention against virus for the general public.

Finally, the threshold of protection considered significant is above 80% filtration. To attain this the researchers introduced

---

[144] IBID Clapp, Phillip W., et al., The researchers used a particle generator to "supplement the chamber with sodium chloride (NaCl) particles that had a median diameter of 0.05 μm (range, 0.02-0.60 μm) as measured by a scanning mobility particle sizer." The results: "Simple modifications can improve the fit and filtration efficiency of medical procedure masks ..."

mask modifications that are totally impractical for general public use, and unsustainable.

This study reminds me of some others I evaluated that layered so many masks over the face of their subject it was seriously interfering with their ability to breathe at all. I will stipulate that if you stop breathing you can eliminate the need to concern yourself with protection from viral infection. But I don't recommend you stop breathing.

What to look for when reviewing studies claiming masks work!

In the course of examining well over 900 studies related to the subject of mask efficacy against a virus, I formed a set of red flags to look for when reading through the literature.

Observational Study versus RCT: We have already shown that the gold standard in scientific research is the Randomized Controlled Trial, and that observational studies are not taken seriously except as exploratory research to help scientists decide whether further research is warranted. No firm scientific conclusion should ever be premised upon an observational study alone. You can legitimately dismiss any study that is a species of what is called *observational science*.

CCP bias: The Chinese Communist Party exerts inappropriate control over every aspect of life in China, including in the practice of medicine. The science does not support masks as an effective mitigation against the spread of a virus,[145] nevertheless, the CCP controlled medical establishment in China supports their use. I think it is a mix of government interference and cultural adaptation. But CCP bias evident in a study is a legitimate reason to

---

[145] Alexander, Paul E., *More than 150 Comparative Studies and Articles on Mask Ineffectiveness and Harms,* Brownstone Institute, December 20, 2021 [ONLINE: https://brownstone.org/articles/more-than-150-comparative-studies-and-articles-on-mask-ineffectiveness-and-harms/ — 11/15/22] For PDF, see Doc. Folder SE035. This study includes important RCTs showing the ineffectiveness of masks.

call it into question. (Note, I'm not talking about *Chinese* influence. There are many very reputable and knowledgeable Chinese scientists. Sadly, many Chinese scientists trained and working in the USA are unduly influenced by the top-down controlled society imposed on China by the Chinese Communist Party.)

Scientism: When a scientist appeals to his own authority as a *scientist* and makes fiat statements supporting a conclusion for which there is no valid scientific experiment, he is practicing a sort of *science* priest-craft. Fauci does this. Remember the bizarre moment Fauci stated that to attack (question) him was an attack on *science* itself. This attitude is not only a display of gross arrogance, it's very dangerous to allow a sort of elite caste system to develop in any field, but also it is especially inappropriate in a field that depends entirely on empirical evidence as its mainstay.

Post COVID (January 2020)[146] versus Pre COVID: I noticed that a flurry of studies attempting to support masks have been produced *post-COVID.* This does not alone disqualify the study, but I noted it as interesting since the results of these post-COVID studies began contradicting western scientific consensus with very weak observational studies and without testing their conclusions by carefully constructed RCTs. Therefore, I recommend you look closely at post-COVID studies purporting to prove masks are adequate for personal and/or community protection from the spread of virus. What I noticed is that after a few attempts at RCTs, it was given up, and *scientists* began shifting toward embracing the observational study approach used in eastern cultures. As everyone knows, these are very susceptible to the influence of cultural, personal, and/or political bias.

Droplets versus virus particles: Watch out for studies that talk about particle size but then switch to discussing droplet size when

---

[146] Katella, Kathy, *Our Pandemic Year — A COVID-19 Timeline,* Yale Medicine, March 9, 2021 [ONLINE: https://www.yalemedicine.org/news/covid-timeline — 2/7/23] For PDF, see OAI120. Katella marks the beginning of the COVID-19 era at January 2020.

it comes to mask efficacy. These studies sometimes openly, but often covertly, admit masks will not block something so small as a virion. What you should watch for, however, is even when they provide evidence that masks can block larger droplets, almost none of these studies addresses the issue of near immediate droplet evaporation. To get adequate information about droplet evaporation, and the dynamics of droplets breaking down upon impact with the mask material, and etc., you must cross reference to other studies, as I have done in my research.[147] In my opinion, any study examining a mask's ability to capture droplets should mention the fact that droplets evaporate very quickly and discuss what happens to the droplet upon impact with the mask, and what happens to the virion as the droplet shrinks and finally reaches full desiccation (complete loss of moisture).

Specious argument: By *specious argument* I mean the many instances I believe some researchers are purposely attempting to fool the average non-scientific reader.[148]

Equivocal conclusions: I noticed that in early post-COVID studies, conclusions favoring mask use were presented in equivocal language, but as we got deeper into the pandemic, the scientists became more forceful in their recommendations for using masks. Nevertheless, you will notice, as I did, within the study scientists have difficulty breaking from their training, and will consistently use language such as *maybe, might, could, perhaps,* and other qualifying language. An empirical study that establishes facts will not present those facts with such language. An example would be when discussing the size of virus particles. Researchers don't bother with language indicating the fact that the conclusion a COVID particle is 125 nanometers is an approximation (the size ranges from as small as 40 to as large as 170 nm). This is because it is an empirically established approximation. Therefore, most are

---

147 See Doc. Folder TECH for several articles addressing these and other pertinent questions.
148 See Doc. Folder OR, examine my notes identified as SP:.

comfortable stipulating 125 nanometers as the size even though the most common stipulated range is 70-140. What this means is that when scientists use equivocating language, they are saying the *science* is still uncertain.

The bottom line is that none of the studies purporting to prove masks work actually do so. A study that demonstrates masks capture 25% to even 80% of droplets that are 200-1000 nm is meaningless. That's because, as I have shown from the science, droplets break down upon impact with mask material and evaporate very quickly into droplet nuclei that will be drawn deeply into the lower regions of your lungs or be launched into the atmosphere as aerosols. A study that *proves* masks reduce the number of virions expressed into the atmosphere from the wearer, but does not take leakage into consideration is tantamount to malpractice. Even if a study claims that a modified mask can capture 80-90% of particles as small as 125 nm, according to the IAH (Independent Action Hypothesis), any one virion escaping capture can transmit a disease. Besides, none of these "modified masks" can be seriously considered for public use. A study that demonstrates adequate mask efficacy can be obtained if you wear so many you can't breathe is ridiculous. Yet, consistently, these are the sorts of studies we are presented as proving masks *can* protect the wearer and/or the community from the spread of a virus.

Chapter Eight:
Where is the outrage?

You would expect a general cry of outrage against the double-talk, flip-flop, and outright science fraud we've been exposed to during this pandemic. Think about it! Beyond the insult to our intelligence from arrogant establishment medical leaders, like Fauci, who admit they lied to us about masks in order to manipulate us, and beyond the fact that these medical professionals, who ought to know better, apparently decided to side with the government narrative against the interests of their patients, let alone the interests of genuine science — beyond all that, what about the lives that have been lost as a direct result of politicizing health care.

For example, the number of lives that honest doctors could have saved if they were allowed to prescribe Hydroxychloroquine and Ivermectin is estimated to be in the hundreds of thousands, or millions.[149][150][151][152] Instead, the government medical establishment, functioning as shills for the pharmaceutical companies involved in this scam, accepted a faked scientific study referenced as the

---

[149] Dougherty, Jon, *Report: Early Covid treatments could have saved thousands of lives, but research was suppressed,* BDP Business & Politics, May 18, 2021 [ONLINE: https://www.bizpacre view.com/2021/05/18/report-early-covid-treatments-could-have-saved-thousands-of-lives-but-research-was-suppressed-1075996/ — 11/17/22] For PDF, see Doc. Folder OAI99.

[150] Mercola, Joseph *Early At-Home Treatments Could Save 85% of Covid Deaths,* The Most Revolutionary Act, July 11, 2021 [ONLINE: https://stuartbramhall.wordpress.com/2021/07/11/early-at-home-treatments-could-save-85-of-covid-deaths/ — 11/17/22] For PDF, see Doc. Folder OAI90.

[151] Johnson, Senator US, *Sen. Johnson: Develop and Offer Early Treatment for Covid Rather Than Slandering Those Who Advocate It,* Ron Johnson, Senator for Wisconsin, PRESS RELEASES, September 1, 2021 [ONLINE: https://www.ronjohnson.senate.gov/2021/9/sen-johnson-develop-and-offer-early-treatment-for-covid-rather-than-slandering-those-who-advocate-it — 11/17/22] For PDF, see Doc. Folder OAI100.

[152] Swart, Nadya, *Covid 19 early treatment — how much damage has been done by ignoring these options?* October 6, 2021 [ONLINE: https://www.biznews.com/health/2021/10/06/early-treatment — 11/17/22] For PDF, see Doc. Folder OAI101.

Lancet study, [153] promoting fear, pretending to prove Hydroxychloroquine is not only ineffective for use against COVID-19 but even dangerous. It was a lie! A fact stipulated by none other than Richard Horton, editor in chief of *The Lancet,* who called the study "a monumental fraud."[154] And it's clear to me that Fauci, and all the leadership in what I have described as the medical establishment, KNEW IT WAS A LIE! Folks; they lied to us on purpose! And their lies cost lives.

A Loaded Statement

Earlier, I referred to "The government medical establishment, functioning as shills for the pharmaceutical companies involved in this ..." That's a *loaded* statement. It requires support to be taken

---

[153] Alliance For Human Research Protection (AHRP) *Updated: Lancet Published a Fraudulent Study: Editor Calls it "Department of Error,"* AHRP, Jun 2, 2020 [ONLINE: https://ahrp.org/the-lancet-published-a-fraudulent-study-editor-calls-it-department-of-error/ — 11/17/22] For PDF, see OAI102. See the following for documentation that Lancet retracted this study when it was exposed as fraudulent: Tristan, Justice *Lancet Formally Retracts Fake Hydroxychloroquine Study Used By Media To Attack Trump,* The Federalist — Health, June 4, 2020 [ONLINE: https://thefederalist.com/2020/06/04/lancet-formally-retracts-fake-hydroxychloroquine-study-used-by-media-to-attack-trump-inbox/ — 11/17/22] For PDF, see Doc. Folder OAI29b. See also The Economic Times, Staff, *Controversial Lancet study linking HCQ deaths in Covit-19 treatment retracted,* June 5, 2020 [ONLINE: https://economictimes.indiatimes.com/news/science/controversial-lancet-study-linking-hcq-deaths-in-covid-19-treatment-retracted/articleshow/76207563.cms — 11/17/22] For PDF, see Doc. Folder OAI103. To see the formal retraction statement: Mehra, Mandeep R., Ruschitzka, Frank, & Patel, Amit N., *Retraction—Hydroxychloroquine or chloroquine with or without a macrolide for treatment of COVID-19: a multinational registry analysis,* June 13, 2020 [ONLINE: https://www.thelancet.com/journals/lancet/article/PIIS0140-6736(20)31324-6/fulltext — 11/16/922]. For PDF, see Doc. Folder OAI84. NOTE: Amit Nilkanth Patel is related by marriage to the founder of Surgisphere, the organization responsible for the infamous Lancet study. The editor in chief of *The Lancet* remarked that the paper in question was a fabrication; he called it "a monumental fraud." Patel reportedly is the author who called for the retraction.

[154] Rosenblum, Yonoson, *When Politics Corrupt Science,* Jewish Media Resources, Rosenblum's Columns, September 2, 2020 [ONLINE: https://www.jewishmediaresources.com/2068/when-politics-corrupts-science — 11/17/22] For PDF, see Doc. Folder OAI104. See also Wikipedia, the free encyclopedia, *Surgisphere,* Wikipedia, page last edited: October 3, 2022 [ONLINE: https://en.wikipedia.org/wiki/Surgisphere — 11/17/22] For PDF, see Doc. Folder OAI105. "Richard Horton, editor-in-chief of *The Lancet,* called the paper 'a fabrication' and 'a monumental fraud.'" — citing "Roni Caryn Rabin (14 June 2020). 'The Pandemic Claims New Victims: Prestigious Medical Journals'. *The New York Times.* Retrieved 18 June 2020."

seriously. I have space for only one example of several available. Consider the following, and you decide.

The FDA sent a letter advising Pfizer on the status of FDA approval of the BioNTech vaccine—a.k.a. the Pfizer shot—then in use, and a new vaccine called COMIRNATY.[155] *Please read the letter*; I linked it below. The letter did not inform Pfizer that their BioNTech vaccine (the COVID-19 vaccine as of August, 2021) was fully approved. The letter expressly stated its use continues under Emergency Use Authorization. *Read the letter.* The vaccine that the FDA declared to be fully approved is called COMIRNATY, and in the letter, it is made clear it was not then available in the United States. Furthermore, the letter contained very explicit trials Pfizer must complete before the FDA would release it for use in America.

Using the above mentioned FDA correspondence as evidence that the Pfizer vaccine had received full FDA approval is outrageous fraud. How is the FDA implicated in this fraud? The FDA has refused to go public and expose the lie repeatedly told by the Establishment Media (aka, MSM), which used the letter to claim the Pfizer shot is fully FDA approved. This is a matter of such importance it is impossible to believe the FDA is unaware of how the establishment media reported on these letters. It is equally impossible to believe their silence in the matter means anything other than that the FDA is complicit in the fraud. Furthermore, it is impossible to excuse the EM (Establishment Media; aka Legacy Media) for their gross negligence and dereliction of their duty. Only

---

[155] FDA BLA APPROVAL, August 23, 2021, correspondence to BioNTech Manufacturing GmbH, Attention: Amit Patel, Pfizer Inc. [ONLINE: https://www.fda.gov/media/151710/download — 11/16/22] For PDF, see Doc. Folder OAI91. This is the actual letter sent from FDA to Pfizer. Also, see this examination of the two letters used to support the lie that the FDA has approved the Pfizer shot: Mining Awareness, *FDA Only Renewed Emergency Use Authorization for Pfizer; Approval was for BioNTech's Cominraty with Years of Additional Safety Studies Required (Thru 2027)*, August 25, 2021 [ONLINE: https://miningawareness.wordpress.com/2021/08/25/fda-only-renewed-emergency-use-authorization-for-pfizer-approval-was-for-biontechs-comirnaty-with-years-of-additional-safety-studies-required-thru-2027/ — 11/16/22] For PDF, see Doc. Folder OAI92.

a fool can fail to see the so-called Legacy Media defrauded the public with disinformation.

As pointed out above, the "scientific" study created to show Hydroxychloroquine (HCQ) was ineffective and unsafe against COVID-19 was fully exposed as a fraud.[156] The truth is that HCQ and other remedies have proved to be helpful. And now we know that doctors could have saved hundreds of thousands of lives if the politicians had not interfered. But we cannot ignore the role played by the establishment government-connected big-pharma doctors who sold themselves to corporate pharmaceutical corporations and, for profit, violated their oath: *primum non nocere,* "above all, do no harm."[157]

Summary Conclusion: A Vote of No Confidence

The people we have entrusted with our health have lied to us. Our confidence in the government medical establishment is broken. And yet, there seems to be little general outrage! Why?

I first began visiting Russia only a year after the Berlin Wall came down. I have a piece of that wall on a plaque with a small segment of the bobbed wire used to discourage efforts to escape the tyranny of Communism. My first visit was for 21 days, and began in Kiev, Ukraine. From there I travelled by train into Russia and Belarus. In Russia, I visited Moscow and St. Petersburg

---

[156] IBID. Mehra, Mandeep R., Ruschitzka, Frank, & Patel, Amit N., Retraction—Hydroxychloroquine or chloroquine with or without a macrolide for treatment of COVID-19: a multinational registry analysis, June 13, 2020 [ONLINE: https://www.thelancet.com/journals/ lancet/article/PIIS0140-6736(20)31324-6/fulltext — 11/16/922]. For PDF, see Doc. Folder OAI84.

[157] Smith, Cedric M., *Origin and uses of primum non nocere—above all, do no harm!* PubMed, National Library of Medicine, NIH, April, 2005 [ONLINE: https://pubmed.ncbi.nlm.nih.gov/15778417/ — 12/21/22] For PDF, see Doc. Folder OAI119. This article is an example of the trend I have observed in medicine away from the ideals that guided us in the past century, toward relaxing those standards, and even removing those guardrails that kept American medicine away from the cliff that tends toward Auschwitz. Smith ponders "its applicability and limitations as a guide to the ethical practice of medicine and pharmacological research," and concludes, "Despite insufficiencies, it remains a potent reminder that every medical and pharmacological decision carries the potential for harm." It seems the doctor finds that maxim quaint. Right! So it would be comforting to know anyone presuming to offer such care would be committed to this *quaint* maxim!

(Leningrad). In Belarus, I visited Minsk. The most tragic thing I learned from talking to hundreds of Russians who lived under Communism was that the people were so accustomed to being lied to by their government, they simply tuned it out. They adapted to life under Communism by developing a cynical culture, characterized by defeatist compliance, and lived in a state of perpetual fear and depression. It was strange for me, as an American, to see how docile they had become. But they were accustomed to it, acclimated to living in fear and depression as a normal part of their existence. That's what is happening in America. The people are so accustomed to being lied to that they are jaded—many have sunk into cynical acceptance! We must not accept, or acclimate to the corruption prevailing in our government and social institutions. We must rise up with moral outrage and denounce the corruption.[158] We must assert our rights, remove these corrupt leaders, and restore confidence in our institutions.

---

[158] The number one most critical issue we must address immediately is election integrity. I'm working on a separate publication that explains the biblical foundation for the truth that governments receive their right to rule by the consent of the governed. Until we get our elections back, we are under tyranny. We must focus on election integrity.

Part Two:
Return to Scripture

Chapter Nine:
Return to Truth / Return to Freedom: Jesus said the truth shall make you free. — John 8:32

Science is about the pursuit of *truth* — what corresponds to what is. Scripture warns us against "science falsely so called."[159] The fact that the Bible refers to a species of science it calls *science falsely so-called* is an affirmation of science *rightly so-called.*

God affirms science! Biblical Christianity has never been at war with *science.* But *science* has developed a very hostile bias against biblical Christianity.[160] Many would say science's war with religion began with Darwinian Evolution and the controversy that arose over introducing that theory into our classrooms. Academic freedom, it was argued, demanded our schools expose our children to this new theory of origins. But where is "academic freedom" now? Honest and well-trained scientists have gathered a significant body of scientific evidence supporting Intelligent

---

[159] 1Timothy 6:20-21 — "O Timothy, keep that which is committed to thy trust, avoiding profane and vain babblings, and oppositions of science falsely so called: which some professing have erred concerning the faith." [Greek terms are transliterated into English.] The Authorized Version is alone in rendering the Greek gno'seos with *science.* All other version use *knowledge.* 1Timothy 6:20 is the only place in the Bible where gnosis [see Strong No. 1108] is found with this ending with epsilon, omega, sigma —English equivalent to e o s. It's an unusual use and form of the word, which suggests a special knowledge derived by personal investigation. The fact that the *knowledge* mentioned in this verse is used in formal opposition to the faith suggests an *academic discipline,* which is how the word was used in 1611. The Spirit here does not have the generic idea of knowledge in view, but a particular use of knowledge, and in this case, a false use. Appropriately, therefore, the 1611 translators selected a fitting word from that time, *science,* which then referred to *collective knowledge,* as that found represented formally in some academic discipline. Isaac Newton was soon (b-1642) to make amazing strides in *scientific* enquiry, while at the time some were using *science* to discredit the Bible. The idea of true and false science was what the translators recognized was in view by the use of this unique word. Using *knowledge* instead of *science* fails to acknowledge the uniqueness of this word as it is found in the Greek text (*Textus Receptus, or Stephen's Text*) and disregards it's special use in the context of 1Timothy 6:20. Of course, it also serves to make the verse irrelevant to what has become one of the most profound attacks on the minds of men in our generation—*science, falsely so called.*

[160] A vital distinction differentiates biblical Christianity and other species of religions that co-op the name. For more on the effort to destroy *Christian America,* see David Horowitz' *Dark Agenda: The War to Destroy Christian America,* and David Limbaugh's *Persecution: How Liberals Are Waging War Against Christianity.*

Design. Yet, government schools refuse to expose students to this scientific information because they deem it religious instruction. Biblical Christians do not demand the many variants of Evolutionary theory be forbidden. They ask only that alternative points of view be allowed free expression. So, who believes in academic freedom today?

Amazingly, well-respected news sources, such as Forbes, advocate against people doing their own research: "You Must Not 'Do Your Own Research' When It Comes To Science."[161] What? Such a statement hails back to the days of the Roman Catholic Dark Ages when they forbade people to read the Bible for themselves but insisted they let the priest caste tell them what it says. We threw off this yoke of bondage long ago, and will we turn around and put ourselves under a new "priest caste" — the *Scientist?*

Some are surprised to discover that the Bible is not contrary to science. But I grew up in a home where the Bible and science were highly regarded. One of the greatest prophets, Daniel, was reputed to have been a man knowledgeable of science (Daniel 1:4). Job is famous for his advanced knowledge of science: millennia before the *modern age*, Job spoke of the Earth as hanging in space upon nothing (Job 26:7). Another prophet, Isaiah, spoke of the Earth as being spherical (Isaiah 40:22)—700 years before the birth of Christ. Moses wrote that the life of the flesh is in the blood millennia before modern science made the discovery (Leviticus 17:11). However, as I pointed out above, the Bible also warns about science *falsely so-called* (I Timothy 6:20).

Science falsely so-called is *fake science.* Like *fake news* has nothing to do with news and everything to do with propaganda, fake science is not about science at all. Fake science is all about

---

[161] Siegel, Ethan (Senior Contributor), *You Must Not 'Do Your Own Research' When It Comes To Science,* Forbes: Science, July 30, 2020 [ONLINE: https://www.forbes.com/sites/startswithabang/2020/07/30/you-must-not-do-your-own-research-when-it-comes-to-science/?sh=4ecd5b21535e — 11/21/22] For PDF, see Doc. Folder OAI106.

pushing an agenda. *Fake news* spins news into a narrative that advances some ideological agenda. Fake science serves the same end. Today, unscrupulous scientists advance *fake science* in the way dishonest journalists do *fake news*. Like the priests of the Dark Ages, they insist we accept their pronouncements without question, and use the coercive tools of government and bullying to enforce their will. But, as pointed out already, the statements of scientists are not science. The rigorous collection of data, forming a theory, and then using experimentation to confirm it, leaving to peers all the information needed to replicate the experiment and confirm the conclusion — that's science.

What do you say? How about let's return to true science. And true science tells us that the recommended masks do not help control the spread of any virus, and in fact, they do more harm than good.

Chapter Ten:
The Biblical Perspective

The American perspective on human rights that has shaped our culture and guided our civil institutions arose from biblical principles and precepts.[162] Our most cherished values come from the Bible; for example, innocent until proven guilty comes from the Law of Moses. And the foundation of our liberties in America, "All men are created equal and endowed by their creator with certain inalienable rights," is based on a biblical view of man. Other notions, like bodily autonomy, freedom of thought, and speech, also are rooted in our Christian heritage. But unfortunately, as our nation moves out from "under God," we are losing these values and the protections they have provided against tyranny. So let's take a moment to consider a biblical perspective on the issue of mask mandates.

God gave us breath!

First, God gave us breath! God breathed into Adam's nostrils and man "became a living soul" (Genesis 2:7). Because man's life originates from GOD, every man has a natural, inalienable "right to life." Upon the same principle, because man's breath originates with GOD, every man has a natural, inalienable right to breathe. For any other man or entity to by force take control of that right, and attempt to exercise authority over it and regulate and restrict it, is a violation of our natural and inalienable rights under GOD. Every man has a right to breathe. Forcing a mask mandate that restricts our natural right to breathe is an infringement of that right, a violation of human rights.

---

[162] Dr. Benjamin F. Morris collected in one major resource over 1000 pages of documentation attesting to this fact: *The Christian Life and Character of the Civil Institutions of the United States,* American Vision, Powder Springs, GA, www.AmericanVision.org. See also, *The Bible and the Bill of Rights,* Dr. Jerry Scheidbach, www.booksatdbp.com

Second, our health, ultimately, comes from GOD. The Bible instructs us what to do if any are sick among us. We are to turn to God in prayer and call the church's elders for anointing (James 5:14). The Bible also affirms the use of physicians (for example, Luke—Colossians 4:14) and natural remedies (I Timothy 5:23). But we must never shift our ultimate dependency from the LORD to physicians (II Chronicles 16:12 — where we read of God's rebuke against King Asa because "in his disease he sought not to the LORD, but to the physicians.")

A balanced approach to addressing our sicknesses includes spiritual and physical measures: we pray, seek the LORD for healing, and discreetly use doctors and medicine. We "trust the LORD" with all our heart. We trust man only in so far as we may be confident he is trustworthy. Therefore, we cannot give away our responsibility to exercise autonomy and discernment in managing our health. We cannot yield to government coercion in this matter. To do so would forfeit personal responsibility for our health, sacrifice our freedom, and remove our body from under the Sovereign rule of our Creator. Jesus taught us to yield to Caesar what is his, but reserve to GOD what is HIS. Our body and health belong to GOD.

Third, our body belongs to God and not to men. He created us (Genesis 1-2)! Hundreds of scripture references show that GOD holds each individual responsible for what they do in their body and with it. Add the many references indicating each person is personally responsible for its care. Furthermore, God appointed us the steward of our body and has not given this power to any other. Therefore, it is the right of each person to decide what measures they will take to answer their physical needs, trusting GOD for the outcome. This is especially true of Christians, whose body God has purchased and made His temple. When we consider the price, Christ's blood, shed on Calvary, our jealousy regarding God's Sovereignty over our body is enhanced! So the believer's body belongs peculiarly to the LORD (I Corinthians 6:19-20; 7:23;

Romans 12:1-2). For this reason, the believer cannot be forced (compelled, coerced) to surrender control over his or her body to any other person without violating his or her conscience and betraying a sacred trust God has given to mankind generally and to His own children particularly.

Please understand what is truly at issue here. Freedom! Personal bodily autonomy and our rights of conscience are at risk. Consider what is at stake: the right to think for ourselves and decide what is in our best interests in our pursuit of happiness. When it comes to mask mandates, it's ultimately about freedom — freedom from intrusion against one of our most personal rights — the right to breathe freely.

Chapter Eleven:
On the Question of Personal Responsibility for Others

I must address the false notion that God requires Christians to allow the government to direct in the manner of fulfilling Christ's command to *love our neighbor as ourselves* and *do unto others as we would have them do unto us* (Luke 10:27; Galatians 5:14; Matthew 7:12).

The argument goes something like this—you must wear a mask to protect others, or at the very least, out of respect and compassion for their fears, you should accommodate them. They tell us this would be doing to others as we would have them do to us and loving our neighbor as ourselves. Another argument is taken from Romans 13:1-6 and 1Peter 2:13. Because the Bible says we are to obey every ordinance of man and that governments are "ordained of God," Christians are obliged to obey mask mandates.

We are responsible to *do unto others as we would have them do unto us.* But those of us who insist we have a natural right to breathe freely would freely yield the same right to others. However, some will say dismissing the argument in this way is disingenuous since the point is that because Christians are under the command of Christ to exercise charity toward others, we should yield to the mandates out of love for our neighbor. So let's take a closer look at this argument!

First, our responsibility to love our neighbor is an obligation to GOD and His CHRIST. No one should presume to prescribe for others how they are to obey Christ's commandment to love their neighbors. It is dangerous to give the government power to decide what we must do to obey Christ's commandment to love our neighbors. It yields to government power over our conscience, intrudes into our private relationships, and puts the government in the place of Christ and His Spirit in our lives. The believer cannot surrender their conscience to the government without displacing Christ.

Give the government the power to decide for the individual what is the right way for people to discharge their responsibility to Christ for loving their neighbor, and you give the government the power of tyranny. Our present case offers an illustration!

Today, the government attempts to direct how we should love our neighbor in response to this pandemic. Since we are concentrating on the issue of mask mandates, consider the folly of granting the government power to decide how we are to love our neighbor relative to the mask controversy.

We have already established that masks do not protect against something so small as a virus. Remember Dr. Fauci's email instructing government officials against wearing masks because a virus particle is so small it passes through a standard mask. But then the same *government authority* says we must all wear masks, without pointing to any proper scientific study supporting the change. In fact, Fauci has never pointed to any study that proves the masks he recommends protect against contagion or transmission. Instead, we get confusing pronouncements. First, we were told two masks work better than one. Then the medical authorities clarified that one was sufficient, after all. Next, we were told masks were to be used indoors only. Then masks were to be used indoors and outdoors. Then we were told no masks are necessary if vaccinated. Those who were dutifully vaccinated hardly removed the mask before being told to put it back on. They told us the cloth masks are not effective, and within a week or so we were told cloth masks are okay. These same experts told us athletes do not need to wear a mask on the field or court, only on the bench? On top of all this, we endured the humiliation of watching our government overlords in public and private gatherings flaunting their disdain for the mandates they put on everyone else. It's an old problem: "Woe unto you also, ye lawyers [*doctors*]! for ye lade men with burdens grievous to be borne, and ye yourselves touch not the burdens with one of your fingers" (Luke 11:46). The current mask-mandate-follies illustrate why we can't give to government the power to decide how we practice Jesus' instruction to love our neighbor as ourselves.

Besides all that, those knowledgeable about the mask issue may rightly argue they do not wear a mask precisely because they love their neighbor.

Finally, only GOD is omnipotent, omnipresent, and omniscient and can intimately know every case. The government medical establishment cannot! When Fauci and other medical professionals make general pronouncements like the vaccines are good for you, they are being foolishly and arrogantly presumptuous. Unless they have examined you and know something about your medical condition and history, there is no way they can support such a blanket statement. It's dangerous for the government to play God. It's perilous when government and the medical profession team up to take God's place in our lives. Remember what happened in Nazi Germany?

Should we allow the government to dictate how we obey God?

To summarize my point about whether we should allow the government to dictate how we discharge our duties to GOD, consider: our responsibility to love our neighbor is, first and foremost, an obligation we owe to God, and the government is not God. The government cannot decide how we discharge our duty to love our neighbor without grossly infringing upon our freedom of thought and conscience. Government cannot know what is best for the health of everyone. Allowing government, or some other person, to take from us the power to decide how we discharge our duty to love our neighbor robs us of our liberty and gives the government tyrannical power over us. Throughout history, every oppressive government advanced its control over the people with the slogan — *it's for your own good.* Tyranny always follows when the government arbitrarily decides what is for the public good. It never turns out to be in the people's interest.

Chapter Twelve:
On the Question of a Believer's Responsibility to Obey the Ordinances of Man and Submit to The Divinely Appointed Powers

The Bible says we are to obey every ordinance of man (1Peter 2:13). Besides, Christians must abide by mask mandates because God ordained governments (Romans 13:1-6).

The Scriptures instruct believers to honor those in power and submit to their authority. We are obliged to respect the *power* as *ordained by God,* and those who administrate this power as *ministers of God.* Scripture warns us that these ministers of God have not been given "the sword" in vain (Romans 13:4). The Spirit speaks severely against those who "despise governments" (2Peter 2:10). So let me begin by stipulating my recognition of the need for and legitimacy of governments, and the necessity that we obey those appointed to exercise its power. However, as you will see from what follows, nowhere does the Bible put government in the place of God.

Christians who think believers have a special responsibility to obey mask mandates on the ground they must abide by "every ordinance of man" have unwittingly accepted a modern twist on an old medieval doctrine called "The Divine Right of Kings." Today, it might be called the *divine right of government.* We need to revisit this heresy.

No human authority is unlimited. When the magistrates passed an ordinance against preaching in the name of Jesus Christ, the Apostles rightly challenged the law saying, "We ought to obey God rather than men."[163] We must resist any ordinance that infringes

---

[163] Acts 5:29. See Acts 5:26-33, excerpted here for your convenience: "Then went the captain [*strategos,* translated *magistrate* in Acts 16:20,22,35,38] ... and brought them without violence ...

upon our inalienable rights because to yield necessarily removes us from under God. No human authority is without limitations. God has drawn the boundary line of those limitations at our inalienable rights and personal sovereignty under GOD. That's where our Constitution draws them too.

Romans 13:1-6 declares God's ordained limits and purpose for government.

First, Romans 13:1 declares, "There is no power but of God: the powers that be are ordained of God." The word *power* translates *exousia,* a Greek word meaning authority or right to rule. God, by Christ, Who is "the image of the invisible God, the firstborn of every creature" created all things "that are in earth, visible and invisible, whether they be thrones, or dominions, or principalities, or *powers*: all things were created by Him, and for Him."[164] (Emphasis added: *powers* translates *exousia.*)

---

and ... set them before the council [Sanhedrin, a *court*] ... and the high priest asked them ... Did not we straitly command you that ye should not teach in this name? ... Then Peter and the other apostles answered ... We ought to obey God rather than men." This religious court had real magisterial authority in these matters. However, some secularist might attempt argue it was not included in the *ordained powers.* But Romans 13 tells us there is "no power but of God," and adds, "the powers that be are ordained of God" (Romans 13:1). Nevertheless, consider God's disposition toward the abuse of *power* illustrated in Acts 16:18-34. To summarize that part pertinent to this discussion: the Roman magistrates of the Roman colony called Philippi, in a rage against Paul's preaching, first beat and then imprisoned Paul and Silas. At midnight, while Paul and Silas were praying and singing praises to God, God sent an earthquake that shook the prison and all the doors opened. The keeper woke, and drew his sword to kill himself, knowing that if the prisoners escaped, he would be executed. Paul cried to him to "Do thyself no harm: for we are all here." The keeper was greatly moved by this, and asked, "Sirs, what must I do to be saved?" Paul declared: "Believe on the LORD JESUS CHRIST, and thou shalt be saved, and thy house." He received Christ, and emboldened by his newfound faith, he removed the prisoners himself, tended to their wounds, and fed them. The next day, the *magistrates* sent messengers to release the prisoners. Apparently, they felt the quake, and realized they had abused their power and were afraid. Paul refused to leave unless those magistrates humbled themselves, and came personally to the prison to release them. When the serjeants reported to the magistrates what Paul said, and that Paul and Silas were Romans, the magistrates feared exceedingly. They came and beseeched Paul and Silas and entreated them to depart quietly. These magistrates violated their oath and executed a penalty upon these Roman citizens contrary to the laws they were sworn to uphold. Paul did not submit to their abuse of power, rather he challenged it, but did so within the law.

[164] Colossians 1:15-16

The Bible says God ordained all *power*; it does not say He ordained all who hold it. Hosea 8:4 clears this up for us: God charged Israel: "They have set up kings, but not by me: they have made princes, and I knew it not." Israel had put persons in positions of authority that God did not choose. God ordained all *power*, but He does not ordain every *person* holding it.

Furthermore, God is the ordaining authority over all *power* He ordains; it is under God's sovereign rule. Indeed, this verse declares, "All power is ordained of God," and says there is no *power* that is not ordained of GOD. In other words, any *person* exercising power in this world is *under God.* There is no government or personality exercising authority that is independent of God's ordaining authority. Any government or governor that is not under the ordaining authority of GOD is, by this statement, declared null and void and without divine authority.[165]

God the Father has turned over to His Son, Jesus Christ, "all power in Heaven and in Earth."[166] By the resurrection of Christ from the dead, God demonstrated "the exceeding greatness of His power to us-ward who believe, according to the working of His mighty power, which He wrought in Christ, when He raised Him from the dead, and set Him at His own right hand in the heavenly places, FAR ABOVE ALL PRINCIPALITY, AND POWER, AND MIGHT, AND DOMINION, AND EVERY NAME THAT IS NAMED, NOT ONLY IN THIS WORLD, BUT ALSO IN THAT WHICH IS TO COME: AND HATH PUT ALL THINGS UNDER HIS FEET, AND GAVE HIM TO BE THE HEAD OVER ALL THINGS TO THE CHURCH, WHICH IS HIS

---

[165] For example, God did not recognize the authority of king Herod to hold Peter in prison (Acts 12:5 ff). When the Angel of the Lord released Peter, the Apostle did not object on the ground of his own teaching, that he was obliged to obey every ordinance of man. Later, when Herod accepted the accolades of the men of Tyre who called him a god, the same Angel of the Lord struck Herod so that he was eaten of worms (Acts 12:23). It appears God cancelled Herod's *divine right of kings* card!

[166] Matthew 28:18, after His resurrection, "Jesus came and spake unto them, saying, All power is given unto me in Heaven and in Earth." The word *power* translates *exousia,* the same word used in Romans 13:1, and Colossians 1:6.

BODY, THE FULNESS OF HIM THAT FILLETH ALL IN ALL." [167] (Emphasis added to bring attention to the fact that Christ has been set "far above" all *principality* and *power* (translates *exousia*) in this world right now, and in that which is to come.)

Jesus has *all power in Heaven and in Earth.* And He has that *power* right now. Jesus Christ is the ordaining authority over all *power* that is exercised on the earth today!

If Christ created all *powers* and *principalities*,[168] and by GOD has been set "far above" all these powers in this world right now,[169] how is it that we are called upon to "wrestle against principalities and powers"? [170] When *persons* in authority use their power contrary to the ordaining authority they lose their legitimacy. Furthermore, entire *powers* (governments) can be taken over by wicked persons, so that believers are obliged to "wrestle against" them.[171]

Satan is no longer "prince of this world." [172] He has been demoted and made "prince of the power of the air."[173] Satan is the "spirit that works in the children of disobedience."[174] The "children of disobedience" are those that reject Jesus as LORD; they deny that

---

[167] Ephesians 1:19-23

[168] Colossians 1:16 "For by Him were all things created, that are in Heaven, and that are in Earth, visible and invisible, whether they be thrones, or dominions, or principalities, or powers: all things were created by Him, and for Him."

[169] IBID. Ephesians 1:19-23.

[170] Ephesians 6:12, "For we wrestle not against flesh and blood, but against principalities, against powers ..." The word *powers* here translates *exousia*, the same word used in Romans 13:1, Ephesians 1:19-23, and Colossians 1:16.

[171] Ephesians 6:10-21, especially verse 12: "For we wrestle not against flesh and blood, but against principalities, against powers, against the rulers of the darkness of this world, against spiritual wickedness in high places." The word *powers* translates the same word translated *power* in Romans 13:1 and Colossians 1:16.

[172] John 12:31; 16:11: Jesus said, "Now is the judgment of this world: now shall the prince of this world be cast out"; and "Of judgment, because the prince of this world is judged."

[173] Ephesians 2:1-2, "And you hath He quickened, who were dead in trespasses and sins; wherein in time past ye walked according to the course of this world, according to the prince of the power of the air, the spirit that now worketh in the children of disobedience..."

[174] IBID. Ephesians 2:1-2

Christ is right now set above all principalities in this world, today! The children of disobedience not only deny that Jesus is Lord, they also deny He rose from the dead—they effectively declare that Christ is dead! By denying Jesus' Lordship and His resurrection, these people disobey the Gospel command to repent and believe on the Lord Jesus Christ.[175]

These disobedient rebels rage against the rule of Christ (Psalm 2; Acts 4:23-31). Satan moves them to usurp the ordained power and turn it against Christ. When this happens, we are called upon to "wrestle against" these rebel powers in our capacity as ambassadors for Christ (2Corinthians 5:20), obeying God's mandate that we submit to Him and *resist the Devil*.[176]

We must understand Jesus Christ has been given *all power* in Heaven AND IN EARTH (Matthew 28:18—the word translated *power* here is the same word translated *power* in Romans 13:1). Therefore, Jesus Christ is the Sovereign Lord over all *power* in Heaven and in Earth making Him King over all earthly rulers.

Second, Jesus Christ puts clear limitations on rulers appointed to exercise the divinely ordained earthly power.

Jesus Christ ordains the *power* (the government authority) to execute His justice on the Earth. Hence, "Rulers are not a terror to good works, but to the evil."[177] But we know some rulers are a terror to good works and promote evil. Such rulers have no authority, neither in Heaven nor in Earth! Christ has commissioned

---

[175] Romans 10:16, "But they have not all obeyed the gospel." In verses 9-13, the terms of the Gospel are laid out clearly: "That if thou shalt confess with thy mouth the Lord Jesus, and believe in thine heart that God hath raised Him from the dead, thou shalt be saved ... for whosoever shall call upon the name of the Lord shall be saved." The Gospel commands us to "repent" (Acts 17:31), and believe on the LORD Jesus Christ (Acts 11:17; 1John 3:23; John 6:29; see Romans 10:9-13). Those who refuse to "obey the gospel" will face the vengeance of God: "In flaming fire taking vengeance on them that know not God, and that obey not the gospel of our Lord Jesus Christ" (2Thessalonians 1:8).

[176] James 4:7, "Submit yourselves therefore to God. Resist the devil, and he will flee from you."

[177] Romans 13:3, "For rulers are not a terror to good works, but to the evil."

rulers to use the divinely ordained power to execute wrath upon those who do evil and praise those who do good. No ruler has the right to use divinely ordained power to support evil and persecute the good.

We find these statements about power being ordained to execute wrath upon evildoers and to give praise to those that do good in the Scripture. Therefore, we must understand the concepts of *good* and *evil* in the context of Scripture. According to Scripture, through King David, "He that ruleth over men must be just, ruling in the fear of God" (2Samuel 23:3). Like *good* and *evil, justice* must be understood in the context of the Scripture in which God made this declaration.

No ruler has authority to be a terror to what the Bible calls good works. Likewise, no ruler who refuses to be a terror to what from the Bible would be identified as an evil work is acting under the ordained authority of Jesus Christ the Lord. Such persons usurp the *power* and, by force, take it out from under the ordaining authority of our Lord Jesus Christ.

Rulers are appointed to exercise the *power* that GOD ordains.[178] God allows us to choose our rulers.[179] Therefore, we must select rulers that He approves. Bad leaders will cause the people to "err, and destroy the way of thy paths."[180] This is the reason the Spirit of God complained that His people had "set up kings, but not by me: they have made princes, and I knew it not."[181]

We may take two essential insights from the above observations. First, although God ordains the *power,* He allows the

---

[178] Romans 13:1; "Let every soul be subject unto the higher powers. For there is no power but of God: the powers that be are ordained of God."

[179] Hosea 8:4; "They have set up kings, but not by me: they have made princes, and I knew it not ..."

[180] Isaiah 3:12, "... O my people, they which lead thee cause thee to err, and destroy the way of thy paths."

[181] IBID: Hosea 8:4, consider how significant it is that GOD, the Almighty, Sovereign over all His creation, would allow men to set up kings without Him? It is a most profound support to the principle of rule by "consent of the governed."

people to put rulers into positions of authority to execute the duties of the *power*. And second, the people must put persons into *power* that satisfy Christ's criteria for leadership. Rulers must be just and rule in the fear of God because the influence of bad leaders corrupts the entire nation.[182]

Remember that God has ordained all power, and He gave it *all* to Jesus Christ, His Son. This includes any *power* exercised over heathen nations—including Muslim, Catholic, secular, atheistic, and all others, no matter what form is used to administrate that power. Therefore, *all* rulers appointed to exercise the ordained *power* must strive to please Jesus Christ the King. The Scriptures outline the criteria for selecting rulers. For a sampling, consider the following statements from the Bible.

What are the Biblical criteria for choosing leaders?

Romans 15:4 and I Corinthians 10:11 inform us that what was written in the Old Testament was written for our present learning. [183] Therefore, the following Old Testament Scriptures present criteria applicable to the New Testament era rulers: Deuteronomy 17:14-20; Exodus 18:21-25; Deuteronomy 1:13; 2Samuel 23:3.

Deuteronomy 17:14-20 offers insight into the character and conduct of leaders fit to rule: 1. He must be a natural born citizen; "one among thy brethren" (v. 15); 2. His dealings with foreign nations must not be for personal profit, nor entangle the people with foreign influences that would lead them away from the LORD (v. 16); 3. He must have a proper family life and not be a lover of

---

[182] Notice that when God declared His intention to remove Judah out of His sight, He said it was "for the sins of Manasseh" (2Kings 24:3).

[183] Romans 15:4, "For whatsoever things were written aforetime were written for our learning, that we through patience and comfort of the scriptures might have hope." 1Corinthians 10:11; "Now all these things happened unto them [Old Testament saints] for ensamples: and they are written for our admonition, upon whom the ends of the world are come."

money (v. 17); 4. Finally, he must be a man that reads and heeds the Bible (v. 18-19).

From Exodus 18:21-25 we find that rulers must be men who fear God, that are men of truth, hating self-serving covetousness.

From Deuteronomy 1:13, we learn leaders must be men known among the people as wise and understanding.

And finally, 2Samuel 23:3 summarizes it well: "The God of Israel said, the Rock of Israel spake to me, He that ruleth over men must be just, ruling in the fear of God."

Jesus offered important guidance: Matthew 20:25-27; 23:11; Mark 9:35; 10:42-44; Luke 22:25-27. Some would limit the application of Jesus' instructions to those who lead the church. However, there is *no power but of God,* and *all power* in Heaven *and Earth* is under Jesus Christ. His directions governing the exercise of authority would therefore be applicable.

The Lord Jesus discouraged leaders from behaving like bullies or tyrants.[184] He taught servant leadership.

If you consider the qualities God demands of leaders, it's easy to see why America is in such a horrible condition.

***Governments forfeit divine authority when they become subversive to the divinely ordained purpose for* power.**

When rulers usurp the divinely ordained *power* and turn the sword that is intended for divine justice against the evildoers and instead use it to persecute the righteous and oppress the people, they are treasonous against the rule of Christ on this Earth.

---

[184] Matthew 20:25-27, "But Jesus called them unto him, and said, Ye know that the princes of the Gentiles exercise dominion over them, and they that are great exercise authority upon them. But it shall not be so among you: but whosoever will be great among you, let him be your minister; and whosoever \will be chief among you, let him be your servant." See also Mark 10:42-44 and Luke 22:25-27. Servant leadership is emphasized: see also Matthew 23:11 and Mark 9:35; — Jesus taught "servant leadership."

Therefore, the people have the divine right to remove such oppressors from their office.

Coming back to our specific issue, mask mandates: we affirm no human authority is absolute, that all *power* is ordained of GOD and under His Sovereign rule, that *all power* has been committed to the present Sovereign reign of Jesus Christ the LORD, and that all mankind is under the authority of Jesus, Who is our Creator, and by Whom we are endowed with certain inalienable rights. Upon this affirmation, we recognize no right of the government to enforce any mandate that violates our human rights. We declare human government has no legitimate power to deprive its citizens of the free exercise of their inalienable rights, including the natural right to breathe freely.

Chapter Thirteen:
What About Peter's Warning Against Those Who "Despise Governments," And His Command To "Submit Yourselves to Every Ordinance of Man"?

Earlier, I addressed how some have distorted Paul's teaching on the relationship between governments and Christians. What about Peter's command that believers "submit ... to every ordinance of man for the Lord's sake" (1Peter 2:13) and his warning against those who "despise governments" (2Peter 2:10)?

A Summary Review of Paul's Teaching On This Subject!

As I pointed out earlier, Paul taught us that God ordained all power, which means all authority is under God, constrained by the stipulated limits He has placed on human government under His Sovereignty. We learned that God gave all this *power* to His Son.[185] Therefore, we are obliged to submit to such authority,[186] as Peter put it, "for the Lord's sake."[187] Furthermore, we saw that the men who exercise this power are "minister[s] of God."[188] Therefore,

---

[185] Matthew 28:18; Colossians 2:15; Ephesians 1:21 — Matthew 28:18; "And Jesus came and spake unto them, saying, All power is given unto me in heaven and in earth." Colossians 2:15-16; "And having spoiled principalities and powers, he made a shew of them openly, triumphing over them in it." And God has set Jesus "Far above all principality, and power, and might, and dominion, and every name that is named, not only in this world, but also in that which is to come."

[186] Romans 13:2, "Whosoever therefore resisteth the power, resisteth the ordinance of God: and they that resist shall receive to themselves damnation."

[187] 1Peter 2:13-15, "Submit yourselves to every ordinance of man for the Lord's sake: whether it be to the king, as supreme; or unto governors, as unto them that are sent by him for the punishment of evildoers, and for the praise of them that do well. For so is the will of God, that with well doing ye may put to silence the ignorance of foolish men."

[188] Romans 13:4, "For he is the minister of God to thee for good. But if thou do that which is evil, be afraid; for he beareth not the sword in vain: for he is the minister of God, a revenger to execute wrath upon him that doeth evil."

their authority is limited to the purpose for which God ordained the *power*.[189]

Anyone exercising *power* contrary to the ordaining authority of Jesus Christ the King is a usurper and has no legitimate right to rule on Earth. Any usurper exercising the authority of divinely ordained power contrary to the ordaining authority should be rebuffed and resisted. Jesus and Paul rebuffed officers that abused their power.[190] It's what Peter and John did when authorities ordered them not to preach in Jesus' name.[191]

Finally, since there *is no power but of God*, we do not recognize any species of government authority that is out from under God. Because no such authority exists, "For there is no power but of God."[192] This justifies Christ coming with all power and great glory to take all earthly kingdoms under His direct command.[193] It's all His! The wicked have no divine right to rule; that's why they "take the kingdom" by force and violence.[194] Jesus Christ will return and

---

[189] Romans 13:3-4, "For rulers are not a terror to good works, but to the evil. ... for he is the minister of God to thee for good. ... for he is the minister of God, a revenger to execute wrath upon him that doeth evil."

[190] John 18:23; Acts 22:25 — John 18:23, Jesus rebuked the officer who slapped Him for questioning the High Priest: "If I have spoken evil, bear witness of the evil: but if well, why smitest thou me?" Acts 22:25, Paul rebuked the Roman centurion challenging his authority, "Is it lawful for you to scourge a man that is a Roman, and uncondemned?"

[191] Acts 5:29, when the "magistrates" commanded Peter and John not to preach in Jesus' name, they answered: "We ought to obey God rather than men."

[192] Romans 13:1, "... For there is no power but of God: the powers that be are ordained of God."

[193] Matthew 24:30, "And then shall appear the sign of the Son of man in heaven: and then shall all the tribes of the earth mourn, and they shall see the Son of man coming in the clouds of heaven with power and great glory." The word *power* here is *dunamis* — from which we get the word *dynamite*. Christ's right to break into Earth from Heaven and take the entire world under His direct command rests in the fact that He defeated Satan on the Cross and the Father transferred the kingdoms of this world from Satan's power to Christ (Matthew 4:8; Colossians 2:15; see Acts 26:18; see Acts 17:30) and the dominion from Adam's race to the Last Adam (Genesis 1:26-27; 1Corinthians 15:45 with Ephesians 1:15-23; especially verse 21, "Far above all principality, and power, and might, and dominion, and every name that is named, not only in this world, but also in that which is to come."

[194] Matthew 11:12, "And from the days of John the Baptist until now the kingdom of heaven suffereth violence, and the violent take it by force."

command all such rebels to be gathered before Him and destroyed.[195]

So why did Peter warn that those who despise government are presumptuous and self-willed?[196] The short answer is that Peter is talking about government ordained by God, not *power* usurped by wicked rebels who hate Jesus Christ the King.

Paul and Peter are in perfect agreement! Indeed, the Scripture cannot be broken (John 10:35).

Paul's teaching on the divine ordination of all *power* (*authority*) in Romans 13:1-6 perfectly agrees with Peter's teaching in 1Peter 2:13-16 and 2Peter 2:4-10.

The Greek word translated *government* in 2Peter 2:10 is *kuriotetos,* meaning dominion, or human governments, including the rulers appointed to exercise their power.[197] Remember that no government has any power God has not ordained. This does not mean God ordains all acts of authority exercised by the government. It means governments exercising any authority contrary to God are illegitimate—they are without power.

Paul said God ordained all power, [198] and those who are appointed to exercise its authority are called the *ministers of God.*[199] This puts all power and all who wield it under God.

Peter and Paul say the same thing about the responsibility of governments.

---

[195] Luke 19:27 In this parable, Jesus describes the circumstance in which we live today, with the heathen raging "we will not have this man to reign over us" (Luke 19:14; see Psalm 2). When Christ returns, all who rejected His reign will be severely punished: "But those mine enemies, which would not that I should reign over them, bring hither, and slay them before me."

[196] 2Peter 2:10, "But chiefly them that walk after the flesh in the lust of uncleanness, and despise government. Presumptuous are they, selfwilled, they are not afraid to speak evil of dignities."

[197] 2Peter 2:10, " ... despise government."

[198] Romans 13:1, "... there is no power but of God: the powers that be are ordained of God."

[199] Romans 13:4, "For he is the minister of God to thee for good."

Paul said the Divine Decree charges governments to execute wrath against evildoers and reward the righteous.[200] Peter said the same thing. After he told us to submit to every ordinance of man for the Lord's sake, he went on to say, "Whether it be to the king, as supreme; or unto governors, *as unto them that are sent by him for the punishment of evildoers, and for the praise of them that do well*" (emphasis added).[201] Nothing in Scripture says Christians should submit to wicked, God-hating, Christ despising rebels when they usurp the divinely ordained power and use it to reward the wicked and oppress the righteous.

Jesus commands His followers to respect authorities that exercise divinely ordained power to execute wrath against evildoers and reward the righteous. We are to honor them, pay their tribute,[202] and submit to their ordinances, even when these authorities are froward (means crooked).[203] We must submit to these authorities. But when human authority crosses divinely appointed lines and limits, we are expressly commanded to *resist the Devil* and *wrestle against his powers.*

Christians must resist devils and the tyrants that are their human agents!

The Spirit commands us to *wrestle* against principalities, powers, the rulers of the darkness of this world, and spiritual

---

[200] Romans 13:3-5, "For rulers are not a terror to good works, but to the evil. ... for he is the minister of God, a revenger to execute wrath upon him that doeth evil."

[201] 1Peter 2:13-14, "Submit yourselves to every ordinance of man for the Lord's sake: whether it be to the king, as supreme; or unto governors, as unto them that are sent by him for the punishment of evildoers, and for the praise of them that do well." Compare Romans 13:1-5, "Let every soul be subject unto the higher powers. ... For rulers are not a terror to good works, but to the evil. ... For he is the minister of God to thee for good. Wherefore ye must needs be subject."

[202] Romans 13:7, "Render therefore to all their dues: tribute to whom tribute is due; custom to whom custom; fear to whom fear; honour to whom honour."

[203] 1Peter 2:18, "Servants, be subject to your masters with all fear; not only to the good and gentle, but also to the froward." While I think this has application to our question regarding civil rulers, the verse here speaks more directly to masters, or, as we would call them, employers. See 1Peter 2:13-18.

wickedness in high places.[204] The word *wrestle* means we grapple, throw down, and resist. And notice that the Spirit repeats the word *against: against* principalities, *against* powers, *against* the rulers of the darkness of this world, and *against* spiritual wickedness in high places. So Christians are at war *against* principalities, powers, rulers of darkness, and spiritual wickedness.

The Bible tells believers to submit to God and *resist the Devil,* not resist God and assist the Devil.[205] Benjamin Franklin, perhaps unwittingly, encapsulated this biblical principle when he recommended to Congress the following motto for the Seal of the United States in 1782: "Rebellion to tyrants is obedience to God."[206] Since Scripture tells us the Devil is the spirit working in and through the "children of disobedience,"[207] then we must resist what Satan is trying to do through them. We cannot yield to their usurpation of the divine power without aiding and abetting Satan's bid to take the kingdom out from under God by force.

Is our warfare limited to the spiritual forces operating behind the men and women who serve him, or do we have an obligation to resist these agents of Satan?

---

[204] Ephesians 6:12, "For we wrestle not against flesh and blood, but against principalities, against powers, against the rulers of the darkness of this world, against spiritual wickedness in high places."

[205] James 4:7, "Submit yourselves therefore to God. Resist the devil, and he will flee from you."

[206] Galles, Gary M., *17 Benjamin Franklin Quotes on Tyranny, Liberty and Rights,* Foundation for Economic Education (FEE), January 17, 2020 [ONLINE: https://fee.org/articles/17-benjamin-franklin-quotes-on-tyranny-liberty-and-rights/ — 12/5/22]. For PDF, see OAI117. See also Goforth, David, *"Rebellion to Tyrants is Obedience to God!" Benjamin Franklin.* David's Newsletter, May 30, *no year indicated, assumed* 2022 [ONLINE: https://davidgoforth.substack.com/p/rebellion-to-tyrants-is-obedience — 12/5/22] For PDF, see Doc. Folder OAI116. Dr. Franklin recommended this saying to be our motto for our national seal in 1782. It was not adopted in favour of E Pluribus Unum (out of many one). Thomas Jefferson used Dr. Franklin's motto for his personal seal. A National Motto for America was not adopted by an official act of Congress until 1956: In God We Trust. E Pluribus Unum was never by any act of Congress adopted as our nation's motto. Former President Obama was wrong when he disregarded this act of Congress and decided, by fiat, that E Pluribus Unum was the original national motto.

[207] Ephesians 2:2, "Wherein in time past ye walked according to the course of this world, according to the prince of the power of the air, the spirit that now worketh in the children of disobedience."

Paul said we do not wrestle against flesh and blood. Doesn't that mean this is entirely a spiritual resistance and not physical?

A *principality* refers to a realm governed by a prince or a ruler. A *power,* in this context, refers to the exercise of authority to enforce compliance with the mandates of rulers. The *rulers* of the darkness of this world refer to the devils appointed to control territory gained by Satan in this world. Spiritual *wickedness* in *high places* refers to the activity of Satan and his angels in and through the principalities, powers, and rulers of the darkness of this world. These spiritual entities act through their counterparts in the physical world.

This is where the spiritual intersects with the physical: Satan works his evil into the world through people under his control. These people are called the children of disobedience (Ephesians 2:2).

When the Bible says, "We wrestle not against flesh and blood," it means we are at war with the malevolent spiritual forces at work through the flesh and blood children of disobedience.

The fact that we do not wrestle against flesh and blood does not mean there is no conflict between the personalities aligned with Satan and those of us aligned with Christ. On their part, they certainly do make it physical. So, let's look at what it means to wrestle against principalities, against powers, against the rulers of the darkness of this world, and against spiritual wickedness in high places.

First, we wrestle *against principalities.* The Bible teaches that Jesus created all principalities and powers,[208] which necessarily

---

[208] Colossians 1:15-16, Speaking of Christ Jesus, "Who is the image of the invisible God, the firstborn of every creature: for by him were all things created, that are in heaven, and that are in earth, visible and invisible, whether they be thrones, or dominions, or principalities, or powers: all things were created by him, and for him. And he is before all things, and by him all things consist. And he is the head of the body, the church: who is the beginning, the firstborn from the dead; that in all things he might have the preeminence."

includes those He commanded us to wrestle against! So why do we wrestle against principalities created by Jesus Christ?

Even stranger, if Jesus created all principalities, why would He come to Earth to "spoil principalities and powers" by dying on the Cross?[209] (The word *spoil* as used here speaks of when a conqueror defeats an enemy and takes all that his enemy possessed into his power.)

In Colossians 1:15-16,[210] the Spirit tells us Jesus created *all principalities.* In Colossians 2:15, the Spirit tells us He "spoiled principalities"—the word *all* is not used in Colossians 2:15. What principalities did Jesus spoil: those that rebelled and pulled out from under God. Which principalities were those?

Jesus revealed to us that Satan was once "prince of this world."[211] This means the world was his *principality*. It was divided into numerous principalities when this prince attempted to defy God at the Tower of Babel.[212] Satan appoints powerful devils to bring these principalities under his control. Daniel identified two: One was called the *Prince of Persia*, and the other was the *Prince of Grecia*.[213] By the time Jesus came into the world, Satan could boast that all the kingdoms (*principalities*) of the world and their glory

---

[209] Colossians 2:14-15, "Blotting out the handwriting of ordinances that was against us, which was contrary to us, and took it out of the way, nailing it to his cross; and having spoiled principalities and powers, he made a shew of them openly, triumphing over them in it.

[210] IBID. See Colossians 1:15-16

[211] John 12:31; 16:11; John 12:31, "Now is the judgment of this world: now shall the prince of this world be cast out." John 16:11, "... the prince of this world is judged."

[212] Genesis 10-11; Genesis 9:1 — After the Flood, God commanded Noah and his families to spread out and replenish the Earth. Nimrod was the first man to make himself a "king" over mankind and attempted to establish what we now call a one-world-government in defiance of God. Genesis 11:4, Nimrod's followers joined him in his rebellion: "And they said, Go to, let us build us a city and a tower, whose top may reach unto heaven; and let us make us a name, lest we be scattered abroad upon the face of the whole earth." But God intervened: "So the LORD scattered them abroad from thence upon the face of all the earth ..." Thus was the beginning of the kingdoms of man.

[213] Daniel 10:20, Gabriel said to Daniel, "Then said he, knowest thou wherefore I come unto thee? and now will I return to fight with the prince of Persia: and when I am gone forth, lo, the prince of Grecia shall come."

were given to him.[214] Jesus came into the world,[215] bound Satan,[216] and spoiled his principalities, taking them away from Satan.[217]

Jesus delivered the principalities from under Satan's power (Acts 26:18), yet the Devil continues to rebel; he refuses to submit to Christ Jesus. He uses the children of disobedience to "take the kingdom" by force.[218] (By the way, this expression, *the kingdom of God*, refers to God's rule in the Earth. Every parable Jesus taught about the kingdom described God's activity on the Earth during the time leading up to Christ's return.[219] So *the kingdom of God* refers to God's work in the world today.) What *principalities* do we wrestle? Believers wrestle against every principality that refuses to submit to Jesus Christ as LORD and sets itself as the enemy of God.[220]

---

[214] Matthew 4:8-9; Luke 4:5-8 — Matthew 4:8-9, "Again, the devil taketh him [Christ Jesus] up into an exceeding high mountain, and sheweth him all the kingdoms of the world, and the glory of them; and saith unto him, All these things will I give thee, if thou wilt fall down and worship me." See also Luke 4:5-8.

[215] John 3:16-17, "For God so loved the world, that he gave his only begotten Son, that whosoever believeth in him should not perish, but have everlasting life. For God sent not his Son into the world to condemn the world; but that the world through him might be saved."

[216] Matthew 12:29, "Or else how can one enter into a strong man's house, and spoil his goods, except he first bind the strong man? and then he will spoil his house."

[217] See Colossians 2:15, "And having spoiled principalities and powers, he [CHRIST] made a shew of them openly, triumphing over them in it."

[218] Matthew 11:12; see Luke 21:14 with Psalm 2:1-4 and Acts 4:25 — Matthew 11:12, "And from the days of John the Baptist until now the kingdom of heaven suffereth violence, and the violent take it by force." Luke 21:14, Jesus prophesied that the children of disobedience would reject Him: "But his citizens hated him, and sent a message after him, saying, We will not have this man to reign over us." This fulfills the prophecy of Psalm 2, "Why do the heathen rage and the people imagine a vain thing. The kings of the earth set themselves, and the rulers take counsel together, against the LORD, and against His anointed, saying, Let us break their bands asunder and cast away their cords from us" (Psalm 2:1-2). Acts 4:25 shows that we live in the fulfillment of this prophecy: the church prayed, "Who by the mouth of thy servant David hast said, Why did the heathen rage, and the people imagine vain things?"

[219] See Mark 4:11-20, where Jesus referred to the parable of the sower and the soil as a parable of the kingdom of God. See also the parables of the kingdom of Heaven in Matthew 13.

[220] Luke 19:12-21, in this parable Jesus described His delivering to His servants His goods and departing to receive another kingdom, with a charge His servants should occupy until He returned. He prophesied that in His absence his "citizens" (the people of the earth) would reject Him and refuse to be ruled by Him. Jesus said when He returns He will judge His servants for their

Second, remember that we wrestle against *powers*. As I have pointed out, God has ordained *all power* (exousia—authority, right to rule), and we are commanded to submit to the power. So how can the Spirit here tell us we wrestle against *powers,* which translates the same word, *exousia*? Obviously, we submit to the divinely appointed power and resist any usurped powers that act in this world out from under God. I'm sure you begin to understand!

Third, we wrestle against *the rulers of the darkness of this world.* The *darkness of this world* refers to the power of darkness (Luke 22:53), Satan, operating in the world. Remember, he used to be "prince of this world." He lost that title, and he wants it back. He works through children of disobedience to accomplish this. He draws them into his power by blinding their minds to the Gospel.[221] False doctrines,[222] vain philosophies,[223] and science falsely so-called[224] are all used by Satan to keep unbelievers blinded and under his power. Of course, it is ridiculous to suggest that we do not resist false teachers or wrestle against their false doctrines.[225] Wrestling against these spiritual forces of evil necessarily involves us in conflict with the children of disobedience that Satan uses to advance his rebellion on the Earth against Christ.

---

stewardship of His goods and faithfulness in their occupation during His absence, and then He will command all who said they would not have Him to reign over them to be brought to Him and slain.

[221] 2Corinthians 4:4, "In whom the god of this world hath blinded the minds of them which believe not, lest the light of the glorious gospel of Christ, who is the image of God, should shine unto them."

[222] 1Timothy 4:1-4, Paul warned that seducing spirits would teach doctrines of devils through false teachers.

[223] Colossians 2:8, Paul warned against philosophy and vain deceit.

[224] 1Timothy 6:20, Paul warned against "science falsely so called ..."

[225] Titus 3:10; Romans 16:17-18 — Titus 3:10, "A man that is an heretick after the first and second admonition reject." Romans 16:17-18, "Now I beseech you, brethren, mark them which cause divisions and offences contrary to the doctrine which ye have learned; and avoid them. For they that are such serve not our Lord Jesus Christ, but their own belly; and by good words and fair speeches deceive the hearts of the simple."

And finally, fourth, we wrestle against *spiritual wickedness in high places.*[226] The *high places* refer to heavenly places. Remember, Satan is now the prince of the power of the air, the heaven in which the fowl fly,[227] and where the sun, moon, and stars run their courses.[228] Satan is no longer prince of this world. Still, he is prince of the power of the air, the headquarters from which Satan launches his attacks on earthly principalities, powers, and rulers. As kings and priests unto God, we have standing before the Court of Heaven (the third Heaven—God's throne room: 2Corinthians 12:2) and we have authority on Earth to command devils and bind them.[229] We have no time to discuss this here. Get my book, *God's War,*[230] where I elaborate on this at length. But the point is, we wrestle against these powers and resist the efforts of men and women on Earth who serve them.

The spiritual forces of Satan operate in this world through their material servants, and the Spirit of Jesus Christ works in this world through His disciples.

It is a spiritual conflict. However, this spiritual conflict occurs in the physical world.

Here is where the spiritual and the physical intersect. Satan is the "prince of the power of the air, the spirit that now worketh in

---

[226] Ephesians 6:12, "For we wrestle not against flesh and blood, but against principalities, against powers, against the rulers of the darkness of this world, against spiritual wickedness in high places."

[227] Genesis 1:20; Job 35:11; Psalm 79:2; 104:12 — Genesis 1:20, "And God said, Let the waters bring forth abundantly the moving creature that hath life, and fowl that may fly above the earth in the open firmament of heaven." Job 35:11, Psalm 79:2, and Psalm 104:12 refer to the "fowls of heaven."

[228] Genesis 1:14-17; Judges 5:20 — Genesis 1:14-17 tells us God set the sun, moon, and stars and in the "firmament of the heaven to give light upon the earth," and Judges 5:20 associates the stars with heaven.

[229] Revelation 1:5-6, "And from Jesus Christ ... Unto him that loved us, and washed us from our sins in his own blood and hath made us kings and priests unto God and his Father ..." And see Matthew 10:1 where we are told Christ gave us "power against unclean spirits, to cast them out..."

[230] Scheidbach, Jerry, God's War: Why Christians Should Rule the World — the case for Christian involvement in every sphere of civic and social life on planet earth, DBP, 2019 [ONLINE: www.godswar2020.com — available as eBook, Mobi, Kindle, or hard copy).

the children of disobedience."[231] This is the spirit of antichrist that John, in his day (late AD 90s), said was "already in the world."[232] The spirit of antichrist works in and through the children of disobedience. Who are these children of disobedience?

The children of disobedience have refused to obey the gospel.[233] The gospel commands all men everywhere to repent,[234] confess Jesus as Lord, believe He arose from the dead, and call on His name to be saved from the wrath to come.[235] God has determined to pour out His wrath on all who refuse to bow the knee to His Son, the Lord Jesus Christ.[236] The children of disobedience are physical, flesh and blood people that reject Jesus Christ as Lord of the Earth.

The spirit of antichrist, the spiritual, works in this world through the children of disobedience, the physical.

By contrast, the children of obedience have confessed Jesus is Lord, believed on Him, and called upon Him to be saved.[237] The

---

[231] Ephesians 2:1-2, "And you hath he quickened, who were dead in trespasses and sins; wherein in time past ye walked according to the course of this world, according to the prince of the power of the air, the spirit that now worketh in the children of disobedience."

[232] 1John 4:3, "And every spirit that confesseth not that Jesus Christ is come in the flesh is not of God: and this is that spirit of antichrist, whereof ye have heard that it should come; and even now already is it in the world."

[233] 2Thessalonians 1:8; 1Peter 4:17 — 2Thessalonians 1:8, "In flaming fire taking vengeance on them that know not God, and that obey not the gospel of our Lord Jesus Christ." 1Peter 4:17, "For the time is come that judgment must begin at the house of God: and if it first begin at us, what shall the end be of them that obey not the gospel of God?"

[234] Acts 17:30, "And the times of this ignorance God winked at; but now commandeth all men every where to repent."

[235] Romans 10:9-13, "That if thou shalt confess with thy mouth the Lord Jesus, and shalt believe in thine heart that God hath raised him from the dead, thou shalt be saved ... for whosoever shall call upon the name of the Lord shall be saved." See 1Thessalonians 1:10, "And to wait for his Son from heaven, whom he raised from the dead, even Jesus, which delivered us from the wrath to come."

[236] Romans 10:9-13; Isaiah 45:23; Romans 14:11; Philippians 2:10-11 — Romans 10:9-13 stipulates we must confess Jesus is LORD; Isaiah 45:23, the LORD through the prophet declared, "That unto me every knee shall bow, every tongue shall swear," and Philippians 2:10-11 clarifies this to mean "That at the name of Jesus every knee should bow ... and that every tongue should confess that Jesus Christ is Lord, to the glory of God the Father."

[237] Romans 6:17, "But God be thanked, that ye were the servants of sin, but ye have obeyed from the heart that form of doctrine which was delivered you."

Spirit of Jesus Christ resides in the children of obedience.[238] Jesus prophesied His Spirit would move through them into the world (John 7:38-39). The Spirit of Jesus Christ works in and through the physical children of obedience. Christ manifests in and through the mortal flesh of believers in this world (2Corinthians 4:11): the spiritual through the physical.

While the war is between the Spirit of Jesus Christ and the spirit of antichrist, each battle is fought out in the struggle between the children of obedience and the children of disobedience.

---

[238] 1John 4:13; 2Corinthians 1:22; Galatians 4:6 — 1John 4:13, "Hereby know we that we dwell in him, and he in us, because he hath given us of his Spirit." 2Corinthians 1:22, "Who hath also sealed us, and given the earnest of the Spirit in our hearts." Galatians 4:6, "And because ye are sons, God hath sent forth the Spirit of his Son into your hearts, crying, Abba, Father." *Abba* is a Hebrew expression of endearment equivalent to our word *Daddy*.

Chapter Fourteen:
You Need to Choose Sides!

If you want to join forces with Jesus Christ against the antichrist forces, here is what you must do.

Recognize you are a sinner, which means you have broken one or more of God's laws. The Bible says all have sinned,[239] and the wages of sin is death.[240] After death, there is judgment.[241] That judgment is hell-fire, followed by eternal confinement in the Lake of Fire.[242] Jesus said none can go to Heaven who die in their sins.[243] To avoid dying in your sin, you must obey the gospel.

Repentance toward God

The first commandment of the gospel is to repent. To repent means to turn from darkness to light and from the power of Satan to God.[244]

To turn from darkness to light means to turn from this world's lies to God's truth. If you are a lover of truth, if you have an honest and good heart,[245] Jesus said you would be drawn to the light of

---

[239] Romans 3:10, "As it is written, There is none righteous, no, not one." Even our good deeds are unacceptable to God: the prophet said, "But we are all as an unclean thing, and all our righteousnesses are as filthy rags ..." Isaiah 64:6.

[240] Romans 6:23, "For the wages of sin is death; but the gift of God is eternal life."

[241] Hebrews 9:27, "And as it is appointed unto men once to die, but after this the judgment ..."

[242] Luke 16:23; Revelation 20:13-14 — Luke 16:23, "And in hell he lift up his eyes, being in torments ..." Revelation 20:13-14, "... and death and hell delivered up the dead which were in them: and they were judged every man according to their works. And death and hell were cast into the lake of fire. This is the second death."

[243] John 8:21, "... ye shall seek me, and shall die in your sins: whither I go, ye cannot come."

[244] Acts 26:18, 26, Paul testified that he preached to the Gentiles the same Message John the Baptist, and our Lord Jesus preached: "that they should repent and turn to God, and do works meet for repentance." This clarified what he meant when earlier in this testimony Paul said, Jesus sent him to the Gentiles "To open their eyes, and to turn them from darkness to light, and from the power of Satan unto God, that they may receive forgiveness of sins ..."

[245] Luke 8:15, Jesus described the "good ground" upon which He would sow His seed as "an honest and good heart." The word *good* here does not speak of moral goodness. It describes a heart that is

God's truth.[246] People hate the light (God's Truth) because their deeds are evil. They prefer to live in the darkness of Satan's lies and deceit so that they can sin without their conscience bothering them. But all that do truth are honest about their sin, and accept God's reproof on their conscience. These will move from darkness to the light.[247]

To turn from the power of Satan to God, you must renounce the spirit of antichrist that works in the children of disobedience. The word *power* translates *exousia;* it refers to Satan's authority or rule. You must renounce your allegiance to Satan and this world and declare your allegiance to Jesus Christ. You do this by confessing with your mouth the Lord Jesus.

Confess, Believe, and Call!

<u>Confess</u> with your mouth the Lord Jesus.[248] Jesus is Lord, and for you to become a child of obedience, after you repent (see above), you must confess with your mouth that Jesus is LORD. This means He is our master, our ruler, and our King. It also means you acknowledge that Jesus is the rightful ruler of Heaven and Earth. All kings (rulers) and kingdoms are under His authority. And it means that there is no authority above His. This confession must be made with your mouth, meaning you must be public about your confession; it cannot be hidden or private. Jesus said any who deny Him before men will be denied by Him before His Father and any who confess Him before men will be confessed before His Father.[249]

---

working properly, where in honesty the sinner will receive conviction in their conscience for their sins.

[246] John 3:21, "But he that doeth truth cometh to the light, that his deeds may be made manifest, that they are wrought in God."

[247] John 3:20-21, "For every one that doeth evil hateth the light, neither cometh to the light, lest his deeds should be reproved. But he that doeth truth cometh to the light, that his deeds may be made manifest, that they are wrought in God."

[248] Romans 10:9a, "That if thou shalt confess with thy mouth the Lord Jesus ..."

[249] Matthew 10:32-33, "Whosoever therefore shall confess me before men, him will confess also before my Father which is in heaven. But whosoever shall deny me before men, him will I also deny before my Father which is in heaven."

<u>Believe</u> in your heart God raised Jesus Christ from the dead.[250] According to the spirit of holiness, Jesus was declared to be the Son of God with power by the resurrection from the dead.[251] Of course, a dead king is no king. Jesus lives! This means He is someone to be reckoned with now and forever. It also means He is able, ready, and willing to forgive your sins. Remember, Jesus warned us that any who die in their sins would not be allowed to enter Heaven.[252] Then He said, "For if ye believe not that I am he, ye shall die in your sins."[253] If you believe on Jesus, He will wash away all your sins.

<u>Call</u> upon His name to be saved.[254] Prayer — calling on Jesus to save you finally expresses your repentance and confession in prayer to God in Jesus' name. God has promised that you will be saved if you call on Jesus' name.

Jesus Christ commands you to repent and believe on Him or face His wrath when He returns to Earth. Join forces with the Spirit of Jesus Christ against the spirit of antichrist. Do it today.[255]

If you have any questions, please contact my office and arrange a time for us to meet, in person or by phone. Go to santamarialighthouse.org and send an email through our contact form. Visit www.godswar2020.com for more information about how to engage in spiritual war for this nation under God. Visit www.brainmassage.net to receive my weekly Brain Massage®

---

[250] Romans 10:9b, "Believe in thine heart that God hath raised him from the dead."

[251] Romans 1:3-4, "Concerning his Son Jesus Christ our Lord, which was made of the seed of David according to the flesh; and declared to be the Son of God with power, according to the spirit of holiness, by the resurrection from the dead ..."

[252] John 8:21, "I go my way, and ye shall seek me, and shall die in your sins: whither I go, ye cannot come."

[253] John 8:24, "I said therefore unto you, that ye shall die in your sins: for if ye believe not that I am he, ye shall die in your sins." (Note: current practice is to capitalize pronouns referring to God. That was not the practice in the 1600s when the KJV was translated. I use the form as it appears in the Scripture quoted.)

[254] Romans 10:13, "For whosoever shall call upon the name of the Lord shall be saved."

[255] Hebrews 4:7, "To day, after so long a time; as it is said, To day if ye will hear his voice, harden not your hearts."

(airs on the radio: AM 1440 (KUHL) / FM 106.3 Saturdays at noon and Sunday mornings at 7 am. The show is distributed as a podcast via Podbean, Apple podcasts, and etc.). Engage with me on my Livestream, Comfort & Counsel For the Present Distress, weekly on Tuesday, Thursday, and Saturday. I usually go live between 8 to 8:15 pm. To connect with my livestream, go to www.brainmassage.net and click on the FB link located at the far right of the menu bar. Come to the Lighthouse. We assemble on Sundays at 9:30 am, 10:45 am, and 5 pm, and on Wednesdays at 7 pm.

God bless you! God bless America! I'll see you in church!

Contact Information

Dr. Jerry Scheidbach

Lighthouse Baptist Church

1310 W. Betteravia Road, Santa Maria, CA 93455.

pastor@baptistlighthouse.org

1.805.714.7731 (Or his personal secretary: 1.805.714.0786)

https://www.brainmassage.net

https://www.godswar2020.com

https://www.santamarialighthouse.org

https://www.facebook.com/brain.masseur

https://www.facebook.com/SantaMariaLighthouse/

Telegram: @jscheidbach; id: 1457144626

TruthSocial: @jscheidbach

Twitter: @jscheidbach; id: 70.109.44.247

LinkedIn: www.linkedin.com/in/jscheidbach

Sarah Green, PA-C

Office: 805.619.7515

Website: (Central Coast Alternative Therapeutics & Rejuvenation) https://www.ccatr.us (Under Construction as of 3/15/23, launch date 2023)

SUPPLEMENTAL Material

To access the more than 3000 pages of supplemental material supporting this research, go to www.booksatdbp.com, click on the *Online Store* menu button, select *Let My People Breathe* (SUPPLEMENTAL Material), and at checkout use the coupon code LMPB-1 to receive all the material FREE.

magistrates, 93, 94, 104

man knowledgeable of science, 82

mandate, 41, 85, 91, 97, 101

mandates, 20, 21, 53, 57, 64, 66, 85, 87, 89, 90, 93, 101, 108

mask, vii, ix, 1, 2, 8, 9, 10, 12, 14, 15, 16, 19, 20, 21, 23, 24, 25, 26, 27, 28, 29, 30, 35, 37, 38, 39, 40, 41, 44, 46, 47, 48, 51, 52, 53, 54, 55, 59, 60, 61, 63, 64, 65, 66, 67, 68, 69, 71, 72, 85, 87, 89, 90, 91, 93, 101

masks, ix, 1, 2, 7, 8, 9, 10, 11, 12, 14, 15, 16, 19, 20, 21, 23, 24, 25, 26, 27, 28, 29, 30, 31, 33, 34, 35, 36, 37, 38, 39, 40, 41, 43, 46, 47, 48, 50, 51, 52, 53, 54, 55, 57, 59, 60, 61, 63, 64, 65, 66, 67, 68, 69, 70, 71, 72, 73, 83, 90

Mayor, 53

medical establishment, 19, 20, 21, 30, 31, 34, 49, 50, 57, 61, 69, 73, 74, 76, 91

microflora, 39

micrometer, 24

Minsk, 77

mitigation, 57, 66, 69

modified mask, 72

morbidities, 29

Moscow, iii, 76

Moses, 82, 85

mosquito, 27

MPPS, 37

MSM, 75

N95, 23, 24, 25, 26, 36, 37, 51, 59, 60, 63, 65

nanometer, 24

nanometers, 7, 24, 25, 27, 28, 36, 37, 44, 59, 61, 67, 68, 71, See nm

nasal cavity, 43

nasopharynx, 43, 44

National Institutes for Health, 54

natural filtration, 41, 43, 45, 46

natural remedies, 86

Nazi Germany, 91

New England Journal of Medicine, 23, 56, 59

NIH, 10, 24, 35, 38, 45, 54, 56, 59, 76

niosh, 23, 24, 25, 26

nm, 7, 23, 24, 25, 26, 27, 30, 33, 34, 35, 36, 37, 38, 40, 45, 59, 61, 67, 71, 72, See nanometers

nonelectret, 68

nose, 26, 33, 43, 44

obedience, 107, 113, 114, 116

www.ingramcontent.com/pod-product-compliance
Lightning Source LLC
Chambersburg PA
CBHW051459250726
48655CB00001B/494